Fetal Alcohol Spectrum Disorders

Fetal Alcohol Syndrome, Pregnancy & Drinking, Symptoms, Cause, Treatments, Prevention

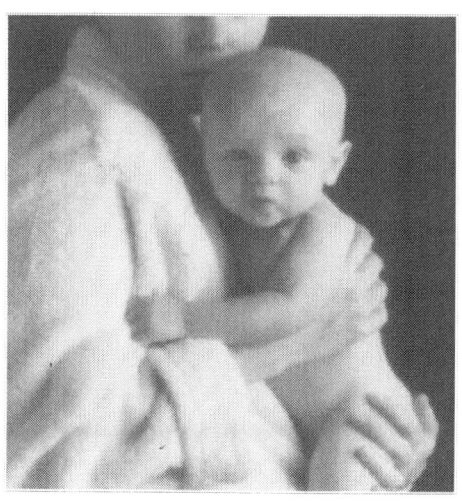

[ILLUSTRATED]

By James Lee Anderson

CONTENTS

INTRODUCTION TO FASD 1
   Fetal Alcohol Exposure 1
   Fetal Alcohol Spectrum Disorders (FASD) 1
   Alternative Names 2
   Transmission of Alcohol 3
   When to Contact a Medical Professional 3

CAUSE OF FASD 4

BINGE DRINKING 5
   Binge Drinking: A Serious, Under-Recognized Problem
      among Women and Girls 5

**PRENATAL ALCOHOL EXPOSURE AND
CELLULAR DIFFERENTIATION** 7

TYPES OF FASD 9

SIGNS AND SYMPTOMS OF FASD 11

WHEN TO SEE A DOCTOR 13
   What You Can Do 14
   What to Expect From Your Doctor 15

DIAGNOSIS OF FASD 18
   Mother's Alcohol Use during Pregnancy 22
   Summary: Criteria for FAS Diagnosis 22

TREATMENTS FOR FASD 23
   Early Intervention Services 23
   Protective Factors 24
   Types of Treatments 25

PREVENTION OF FASD 32

LIVING WITH FASD **34**
  FAS/FASD through the Lifespan 35
  Strategies for Living 35
  More Tips 38

REAL STORIES FROM PEOPLE LIVING WITH FASD **40**
  Melissa's Story 40
  Frances's Story 42

RESEARCH ON FASD **44**
  Understanding and Improving Health Messages about
    Alcohol and Pregnancy 46
  The Consequences of Prenatal Alcohol Exposure 48
  Dysregulation of microRNA Expression and Function
    Contributes to the Etiology of Fetal Alcohol
    Spectrum Disorders 51

**DISTINGUISHING BETWEEN ADHD & FASD IN
  CHILDREN** **62**
  Attention Deficit Hyperactivity Disorder 62
  Fetal Alcohol Spectrum Disorders 63
  Attention and Hyperactivity Problems in FASD 65
  Rationale for Distinguishing between ADHD and FASD 65
  ADHD and FASD 66
  Diagnosis of the Impulsive, Hyperactive, or Inattentive Child 71
  Treatment of ADHD in FASD 72

TIMELINE: FETAL ALCOHOL SPECTRUM DISORDERS 76
  Yesterday 76
  Today 77
  Tomorrow 79

BIBLIOGRAPHY **83**

INTRODUCTION TO FASD

Fetal Alcohol Exposure

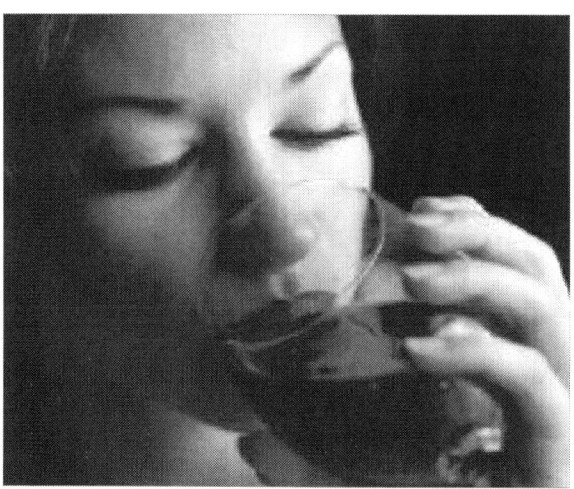

Fetal alcohol exposure occurs when a woman drinks while pregnant. No amount of alcohol is safe for pregnant women to drink. Nevertheless, data from prenatal clinics and postnatal studies suggest that 20 to 30 percent of women do drink at some time during pregnancy.

Alcohol can disrupt fetal development at any stage during a pregnancy–including at the earliest stages and before a woman knows she is pregnant. Research shows that binge drinking, which means consuming four or more drinks per occasion, and regular heavy drinking put a fetus at the greatest risk for severe problems.

Fetal Alcohol Spectrum Disorders (FASD)

Drinking during pregnancy can cause brain damage, leading to a range of developmental, cognitive, and behavioral problems, which can appear at any time during childhood. Fetal Alcohol Spectrum Disorders (FASD) is the umbrella term for the different diagnoses, which include Fetal Alcohol Syndrome, partial Fetal Alcohol Syndrome, Alcohol-related neurodevelopmental disorder, and Alcohol-related birth defects.

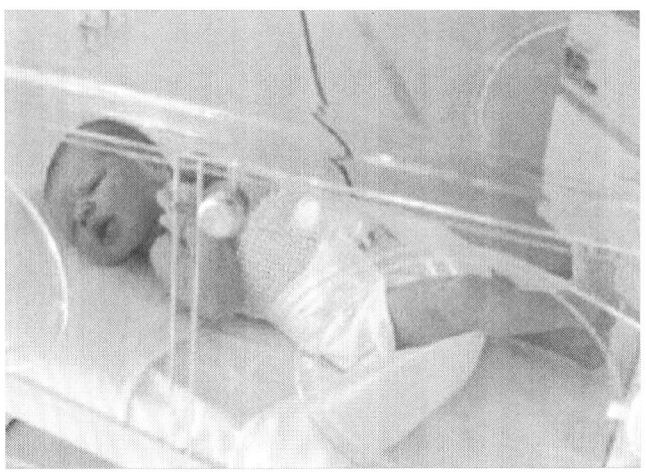

People with FASD often have difficulty in the following areas:

- Coordination
- Emotional control
- School work
- Socialization
- Holding a job

In addition, they often make bad decisions, repeat the same mistakes, trust the wrong people, and do not understand the consequences of their actions.

Alternative Names

Alcohol in Pregnancy; Alcohol-Related Birth Defects (ARBD); Fetal Alcohol Effects (FAE); Fetal Alcohol Syndrome (FAS); Alcohol-Related Neurodevelopmental Disorder (ARND)

Transmission of Alcohol

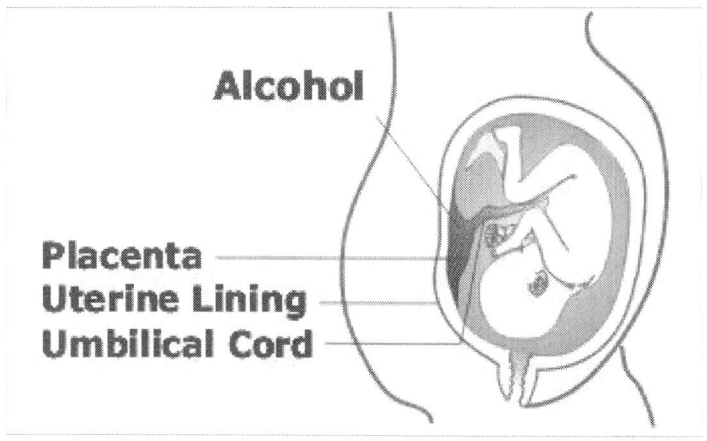

Transmission of alcohol from a pregnant woman to a fetus.

Drinking at any time during pregnancy can harm the fetus. The figure depicts developing parts and systems in the body of a fetus. These body parts and systems represent some of the sites that may be affected by alcohol.

Alcohol can harm your baby at any stage during a pregnancy. That includes the earliest stages before you even know you are pregnant.

When to Contact a Medical Professional

Call for an appointment with your health care provider if you are drinking alcohol regularly or heavily, and are finding it difficult to cut back or stop. Also, call if you are drinking alcohol in any amount while you are pregnant or trying to get pregnant.

CAUSE OF FASD

Using or abusing alcohol during pregnancy can cause the same risks as using alcohol in general. However, it poses extra risks to the unborn baby. When a pregnant woman drinks alcohol, it easily passes across the placenta to the fetus. Because of this, drinking alcohol can harm the baby's development.

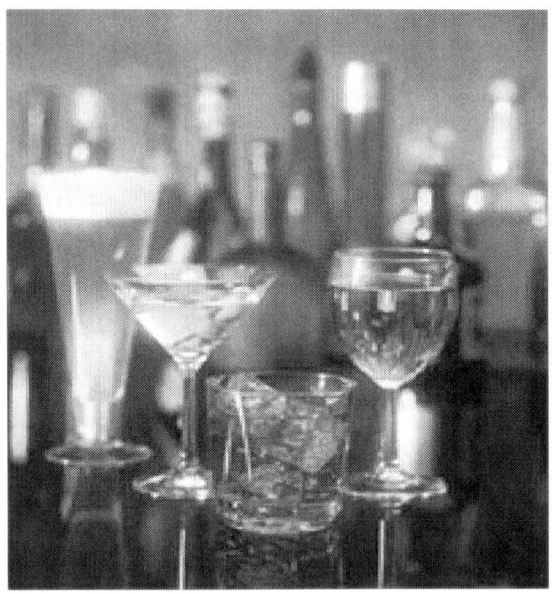

A pregnant woman who drinks any amount of alcohol is at risk for having a child with fetal alcohol syndrome. **No "safe" level of alcohol use during pregnancy has been established.** Larger amounts of alcohol appear to increase the problems. Binge drinking is more harmful than drinking small amounts of alcohol.

Timing of alcohol use during pregnancy is also important. Alcohol use appears to be the most harmful during the first 3 months of pregnancy; however, drinking alcohol *any time* during pregnancy can be harmful.

BINGE DRINKING

Binge Drinking: A Serious, Under-Recognized Problem among Women and Girls

Binge drinking is a dangerous behavior but is not widely recognized as a women's health problem. Drinking too much – including binge drinking* - results in about 23,000 deaths in women and girls each year. Binge drinking increases the chances of breast cancer, heart disease, sexually transmitted diseases, unintended pregnancy, and many other health problems. Drinking during pregnancy can lead to sudden infant death syndrome and fetal alcohol spectrum disorders.

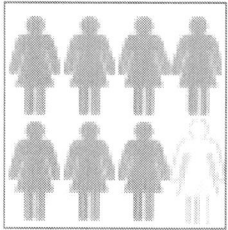

1 in 8
Nearly 14 million US women binge drink about 3 times a month.

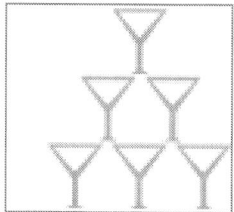

Women average 6 drinks per binge.

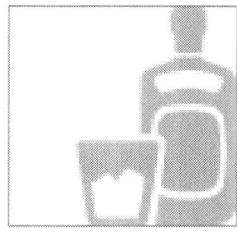

1 in 5 high school girls binge drink.

About 1 in 8 women aged 18 years and older and 1 in 5 high school girls binge drink. Women who binge drink do so frequently – about 3 times a month – and have about 6 drinks per binge. There are effective actions communities can take to prevent binge drinking among women and girls.

*Binge drinking for women is defined as consuming 4 or more alcohol drinks (beer, wine, or liquor) on an occasion.

PRENATAL ALCOHOL EXPOSURE AND CELLULAR DIFFERENTIATION

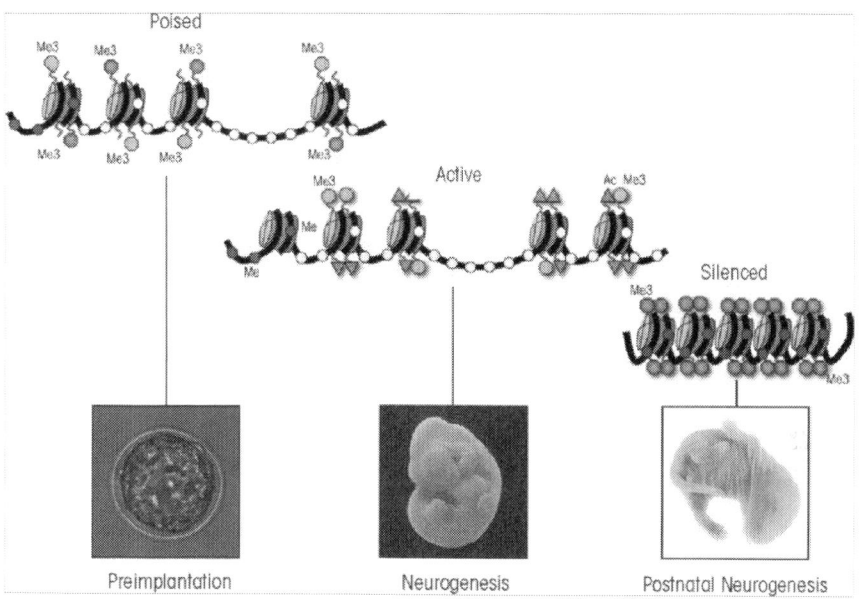

During development of the nervous system, many genes controlling neural patterning are held in a poised or bivalent conformation during early embryogenesis, resolve towards the active conformation during neural patterning, and are silenced during postnatal life. Repression (i.e., trimethylation of histone 3 lysine 27 [H3K27me3]) is imposed by the polycomb group proteins (PcG) (small red circles), whereas activation H3K4me3 is imparted by the mammalian homologues of the trithorax group proteins (TrxG) (green triangles). Correct biochemical function of these proteins and the coordination of the marks they impart are essential to mammalian neurogenesis.

Exposure to alcohol significantly alters the developmental trajectory of progenitor cells and fundamentally compromises tissue formation (i.e., histogenesis). Emerging research suggests that ethanol can impair mammalian development by interfering with the execution of molecular programs governing differentiation. For example, ethanol exposure disrupts cellular migration, changes cell–cell interactions, and alters growth factor signaling pathways. Additionally, ethanol can alter epigenetic mechanisms controlling gene expression. Normally, lineage-specific regulatory factors (i.e., transcription factors) establish the transcriptional networks of each new cell type; the cell's identity then is maintained through epigenetic alterations in the way in which the DNA encoding each gene becomes packaged within the chromatin. Ethanol exposure can induce epigenetic changes that do not induce genetic mutations but nonetheless alter the course of fetal development and result in a large array of patterning defects. Two crucial enzyme complexes—the Polycomb and Trithorax proteins—are central to the epigenetic programs controlling the intricate balance between self-renewal and the execution of cellular differentiation, with diametrically opposed functions. Prenatal ethanol exposure may disrupt the functions of these two enzyme complexes, altering a crucial aspect of mammalian differentiation. Characterizing the involvement of Polycomb and Trithorax group complexes in the etiology of fetal alcohol spectrum disorders will undoubtedly enhance understanding of the role that epigenetic programming plays in this complex disorder.

Exposure of the developing embryo and fetus to alcohol can have profound adverse effects on physical, behavioral, and cognitive development. The resulting deficits collectively have been termed fetal alcohol spectrum disorders (FASD). They range in severity from mild cognitive deficits to a well-defined syndrome (i.e., fetal alcohol syndrome [FAS]), which is broadly characterized by low birth weight, distinctive craniofacial malformations, smaller-than-normal head size (i.e., microcephaly), and central nervous system dysfunction (Riley et al. 2011). The mechanisms underlying ethanol's harmful effects on development are not yet fully understood. Studies in recent years have indicated that epigenetic mechanisms may play a role in the etiology of FASD. This article describes the proposed roles of epigenetic mechanisms in FASD and cell differentiation in general and introduces two protein complexes that are hypothesized to play central roles in these events.

TYPES OF FASD

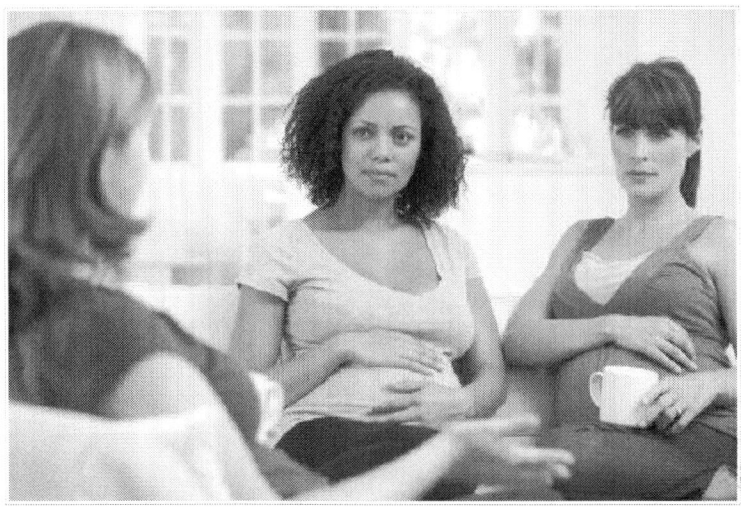

Different terms are used to describe FASDs, depending on the type of symptoms.

- **Fetal Alcohol Syndrome (FAS):** FAS represents the severe end of the FASD spectrum. Fetal death is the most extreme outcome from drinking alcohol during pregnancy. People with FAS might have abnormal facial features, growth problems, and central nervous system (CNS) problems. People with FAS can have problems with learning, memory, attention span, communication, vision, or hearing. They might have a mix of these problems. People with FAS often have a hard time in school and trouble getting along with others.

- **Alcohol-Related Neurodevelopmental Disorder (ARND):** People with ARND might have intellectual disabilities and problems with behavior and learning. They might do poorly in school and have difficulties with math, memory, attention, judgment, and poor impulse control.

- **Alcohol-Related Birth Defects (ARBD):** People with ARBD might have problems with the heart, kidneys, or bones or with hearing. They might have a mix of these.

The term fetal alcohol effects (FAE) was previously used to describe intellectual disabilities and problems with behavior and learning in a person whose mother drank alcohol during pregnancy. In 1996, the Institute of Medicine (IOM) replaced FAE with the terms alcohol-related neurodevelopmental disorder (ARND) and alcohol-related birth defects (ARBD).

SIGNS AND SYMPTOMS OF FASD

FASDs refer to the whole range of effects that can happen to a person whose mother drank alcohol during pregnancy. These conditions can affect each person in different ways, and can range from mild to severe.

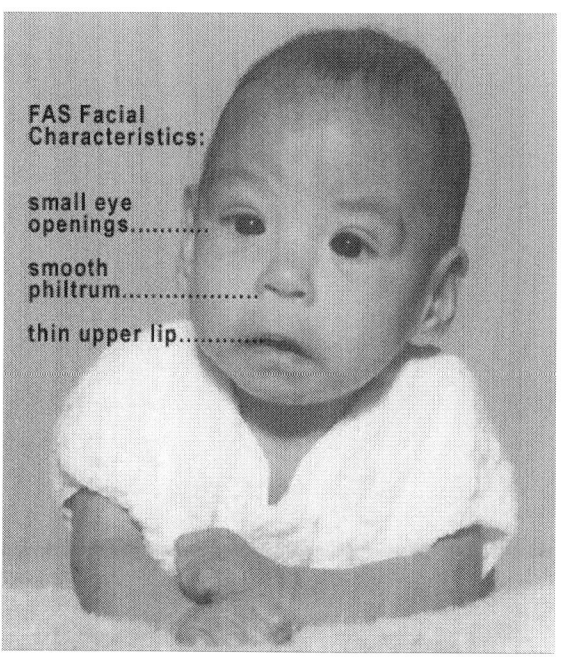

Facial features associated with FASD

A person with an FASD might have:

- Abnormal facial features, such as a smooth ridge between the nose and upper lip (this ridge is called the philtrum)
- Small head size
- Shorter-than-average height
- Low body weight
- Poor coordination

- Hyperactive behavior
- Difficulty paying attention
- Poor memory
- Difficulty in school (especially with math)
- Learning disabilities
- Speech and language delays
- Intellectual disability or low IQ
- Poor reasoning and judgment skills
- Sleep and sucking problems as a baby
- Vision or hearing problems
- Problems with the heart, kidneys, or bones

WHEN TO SEE A DOCTOR

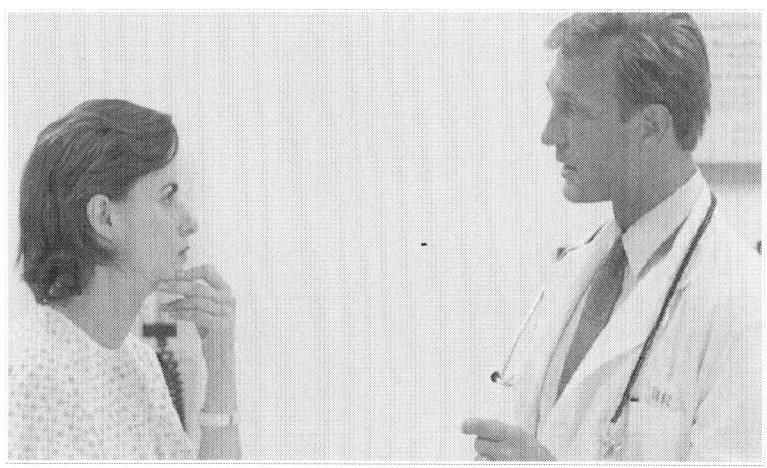

If you're pregnant and can't stop drinking, ask your obstetrician or other health care provider for help.

Because early diagnosis may help reduce the risk of long-term problems for children with FAS, let your child's doctor know if you drank alcohol while you were pregnant. Don't wait for problems to arise before seeking help.

If you've adopted a child or are providing foster care, you may not know if your child's biological mother drank alcohol while pregnant — and it may not initially occur to you that your child may have fetal alcohol syndrome. However, if your child has learning and behavioral problems, talk with your child's doctor so that the underlying cause might be identified.

When you're pregnant and drink alcohol, it enters your bloodstream and reaches your developing fetus by crossing the placenta. Because a fetus metabolizes alcohol more slowly than an adult does, your developing baby's blood alcohol concentrations are higher than those in your body. Alcohol also interferes with the delivery of oxygen and optimal nutrition to your baby's developing tissues and organs, including the brain.

The more you drink while pregnant, the greater the risk to your unborn baby. The risk is present at any time during pregnancy. However, impairment of facial features, the heart and other organs, including the bones, and the central nervous system may occur as a result of drinking alcohol during the first trimester. That's when these parts of the fetus are in key stages of development. In the early weeks of the first trimester, many women may not be aware that they're pregnant.

Although doctors aren't sure how much alcohol you'd have to drink to place your baby at risk, they do know that the more you drink, the greater the chance of problems. Because there's no known safe amount of alcohol consumption during pregnancy, don't drink alcohol if you are or think you are pregnant or you're attempting to become pregnant. You could put your baby at risk even before you realize you're pregnant.

Call your child's doctor for an appointment if you see any symptoms that concern you. Your child's doctor will let you know if your child needs to see a specialist, such as a doctor specializing in heart problems (cardiologist) if your child has a heart issue.

Because appointments can be brief, and there's often a lot of ground to cover, it's a good idea to arrive well prepared. Here's some information to help you get ready for your appointment, and what to expect from your doctor.

What You Can Do

- **Write down any symptoms you've noticed in your child,** including any that may seem unrelated to the reason for which you scheduled the appointment.

- **Make a list of all medications,** vitamins or supplements that you took during pregnancy. Also, let your child's doctor know if you drank alcohol during your pregnancy, and if so, how much and how often.

- **Consider asking a family member or friend to come with you.** Sometimes it can be difficult to remember all of the information provided to you during an appointment, especially if you've been told that there may be something wrong with your child. Someone who accompanies you may remember something that you missed or forgot.

- **Write down questions to ask your doctor.**

Preparing a list of questions can help you make the most of your time with your child's doctor. For fetal alcohol syndrome, some basic questions to ask your doctor include:

- What's the most likely cause of my child's symptoms?
- Are there other possible causes for these symptoms?
- What kinds of tests does he or she need? Do these tests require any special preparation?
- Will my child's condition improve over time? Will it get worse?
- What treatments are available, and which do you recommend?
- How can I prevent this from happening in future pregnancies?
- Are there any brochures or other printed material that I can take with me? What websites do you recommend?
- Are there medications that may help, and are there medications that should be avoided?

In addition to the questions that you've prepared to ask your child's doctor, don't hesitate to ask any additional questions that may occur to you during your appointment.

What to Expect From Your Doctor

Your child's doctor is likely to ask you a number of questions. Being ready to answer them may reserve time to go over points you want to spend more time on. Your doctor may ask:

- When did you first notice your child's symptoms?
- Have these symptoms been continuous or are they only occasional?
- Does anything seem to improve the symptoms?
- What, if anything, appears to worsen the symptoms?
- Did you have any problems during your pregnancy?
- Did you drink alcohol while you were pregnant? If yes, how much and how often?
- Did you use any illegal drugs during your pregnancy?

Although doctors can't diagnose fetal alcohol syndrome before a baby is born, they can assess the health of mother and baby during pregnancy. If you report the timing and amount of alcohol consumption, your obstetrician or other health care provider can help determine the risk of fetal alcohol syndrome.

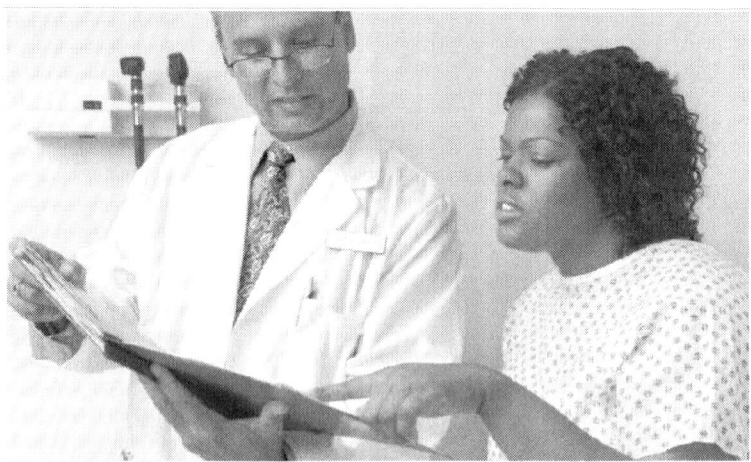

If you let your child's doctor know that you drank alcoholic beverages during your pregnancy, he or she can watch for signs and symptoms of this syndrome in your child's initial weeks, months and years of life. To make a diagnosis, doctors will assess:

- Growth
- Facial features

- Heart health
- Hearing
- Vision
- Cognitive ability
- Language development
- Motor skills
- Behavior

Doctors may refer a child with possible fetal alcohol syndrome to a medical genetics specialist to rule out other disorders with similar signs and symptoms.

If one child in your family is diagnosed with fetal alcohol syndrome, it's important to evaluate his or her siblings to determine whether they also have fetal alcohol syndrome.

DIAGNOSIS OF FASD

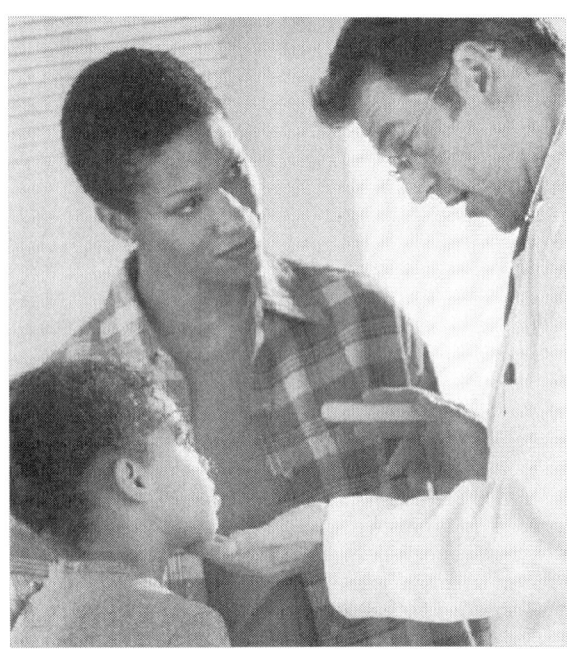

Diagnosing Fetal Alcohol Syndrome can be hard because there is no medical test, like a blood test, for it. And other disorders, such as ADHD (attention-deficit/hyperactivity disorder) and Williams syndrome, have some symptoms like FAS.

To diagnose FAS, doctors look for:

- Abnormal facial features (e.g., smooth ridge between nose and upper lip)

- Lower-than-average height, weight, or both

- Central nervous system problems (e.g., small head size, problems with attention and hyperactivity, poor coordination)

- Prenatal alcohol exposure; although confirmation is not required to make a diagnosis

Deciding if a child has FAS takes several steps. There is no one test to diagnose FAS, and many other disorders can have similar symptoms.

Healthcare professionals look for the following signs and symptoms when diagnosing FAS:

1. **Abnormal facial features.** A person with FAS has three distinct facial features:

    - Smooth ridge between the nose and upper lip (smooth philtrum)

    - Thin upper lip

    - Short distance between the inner and outer corners of the eyes, giving the eyes a wide-spaced appearance.

2. **Growth problems.** Children with FAS have height, weight, or both that are lower than normal (at or below the 10th percentile). These growth issues might occur even before birth. For some children with FAS, growth problems resolve themselves early in life.

3. **Central nervous system problems.** The central nervous system is made up of the brain and spinal cord. It controls all the workings of the body. When something goes wrong with a part of the nervous system, a person can have trouble moving, speaking, or learning. He or she can also have problems with memory, senses, or social skills. There are three categories of central nervous system problems:

    I. **Structural.** FAS can cause differences in the structure of the brain. Signs of structural differences are:

- Smaller-than-normal head size for the person's overall height and weight (at or below the 10th percentile).

- Significant changes in the structure of the brain as seen on brain scans such as MRIs or CT scans.

II. **Neurologic.** There are problems with the nervous system that cannot be linked to another cause. Examples include poor coordination, poor muscle control, and problems with sucking as a baby.

III. **Functional.** The person's ability to function is well below what's expected for his or her age, schooling, or circumstances. To be diagnosed with FAS, a person must have:

- Cognitive deficits (e.g., low IQ), or significant developmental delay in children who are too young for an IQ assessment.

or

- Problems in at least three of the following areas:

    a. **Cognitive deficits (e.g., low IQ) or developmental delays.** Examples include specific learning disabilities (especially math), poor grades in school, performance differences between verbal and nonverbal skills, and slowed movements or reactions.

    b. **Executive functioning deficits.** These deficits involve the thinking processes that help a person manage life tasks. Such deficits include poor organization and planning, lack of inhibition, difficulty grasping cause and effect, difficulty following multistep directions, difficulty doing things in a new way or thinking of things in a new way, poor judgment, and inability to apply knowledge to new situations.

c. **Motor functioning delays.** These delays affect how a person controls his or her muscles. Examples include delay in walking (gross motor skills), difficulty writing or drawing (fine motor skills), clumsiness, balance problems, tremors, difficulty coordinating hands and fingers (dexterity), and poor sucking in babies.

d. **Attention problems or hyper-activity.** A child with these problems might be described as "busy," overly active, inattentive, easily distracted, or having difficulty calming down, completing tasks, or moving from one activity to the next. Parents might report that their child's attention changes from day to day (e.g., "on" and "off" days).

e. **Problems with social skills.** A child with social skills problems might lack a fear of strangers, be easily taken advantage of, prefer younger friends, be immature, show inappropriate sexual behaviors, and have trouble understanding how others feel.

f. **Other problems.** Other problems can include sensitivity to taste or touch, difficulty reading facial expression, and difficulty responding appropriately to common parenting practices (e.g., not understanding cause-and-effect discipline)

Mother's Alcohol Use during Pregnancy

Confirmed alcohol use during pregnancy can strengthen the case for FAS diagnosis. Confirmed absence of alcohol exposure would rule out the FAS diagnosis. It's helpful to know whether or not the person's mother drank alcohol during pregnancy. But confirmed alcohol use during pregnancy is not needed if the child meets the other criteria.

Summary: Criteria for FAS Diagnosis

A diagnosis of FAS requires the presence of all three of the following findings:

1. All three facial features

2. Growth deficits

3. Central nervous system problems. A person could meet the central nervous system criteria for FAS diagnosis if there is a problem with the brain structure, even if there are no signs of functional problems.

TREATMENTS FOR FASD

CDC has provided the information on this page because it may be of interest to you. CDC does not necessarily endorse the views or information presented. CDC cannot answer personal medical questions. Please talk to your health care professional about specific questions concerning appropriate care, treatment, or other medical advice.

No two people with an FASD are exactly alike. FASDs can include physical or intellectual disabilities, as well as problems with behavior and learning. These symptoms can range from mild to severe. Treatment services for people with FASDs should be different for each person depending on the symptoms.

Early Intervention Services

There is no cure for FASDs, but research shows that early intervention treatment services can improve a child's development. Early intervention services help children from birth to 3 years of age (36 months) learn important skills. Services include therapy to help the child talk, walk, and interact with others. Therefore, it is important to talk to your child's doctor as soon as possible if you think your child has an FASD or other developmental problem.

Even if your child has not received a diagnosis, he or she might qualify for early intervention treatment services. The **Individuals with Disabilities Education Act (IDEA)** says that children younger than 3 years of age who are at risk of having developmental delays may be eligible for services. The early intervention system in your state will help you have your child evaluated and provide services if your child qualifies.

In addition, treatment for particular symptoms, such as speech therapy for language delays, often does not need to wait for a formal diagnosis.

Protective Factors

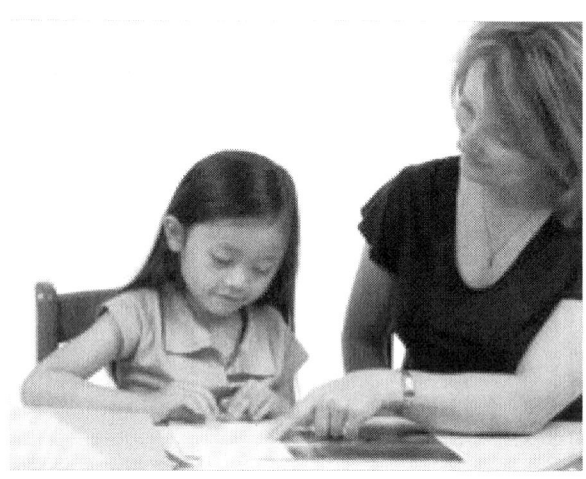

Studies have shown that some protective factors can help reduce the effects of FASDs and help people with these conditions reach their full potential. Protective factors include:

- **Early diagnosis.** A child who is diagnosed at a young age can be placed in appropriate educational classes and get the social services needed to help the child and his or her family. Early diagnosis also helps families and school staff to understand why the child might act or react differently from other children sometimes.

- **Involvement in special education and social services.** Children who receive special education geared towards their specific needs and learning style are more likely to reach their full potential. Children with FASDs have a wide range of behaviors and challenges that might need to be addressed. Special education programs can better meet each child's needs. In addition, families of children with FASDs who receive social services, such as counseling or respite care have more positive experiences than families who do not receive such services.

- **Loving, nurturing, and stable home environment.** Children with FASDs can be more sensitive than other children to disruptions, changes in lifestyle or routines, and harmful relationships. Therefore, having a loving, stable home life is very important for a child with an FASD. In addition, community and family support can help prevent secondary conditions, such as criminal behavior, unemployment, and incomplete education.

- **Absence of violence.** People with FASDs who live in stable, non-abusive households or who do not become involved in youth violence are much less likely to develop secondary conditions than children who have been exposed to violence in their lives. Children with FASDs need to be taught other ways of showing their anger or frustration.

Types of Treatments

Many types of treatments are available for people with FASDs. They can generally be broken down into five categories:

- Medical Care
- Medication
- Behavior and Education Therapy
- Parent Training
- Alternative Approaches

Medical Care

People with FASDs have the same health and medical needs as people without FASDs. Like everyone else, they need well-baby care, vaccinations, good nutrition, exercise, hygiene, and basic medical care. But, for people with FASDs, concerns specific to the disorder must also be monitored and addressed either by a current doctor or through referral to a specialist. The types of treatments needed will be different for each person and depend upon the person's symptoms.

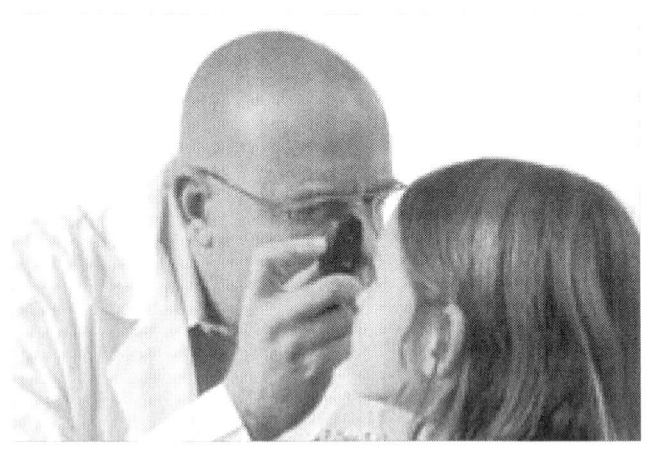

Types of medical specialists might include:

- Pediatrician
- Primary care provider
- Dysmorphologist
- Otolaryngologist
- Audiologist
- Immunologist
- Neurologist
- Mental health professionals (child psychiatrist and psychologist, school psychologist, behavior management specialist)
- Ophthalmologist
- Plastic surgeon
- Endocrinologist
- Gastroenterologist
- Nutritionist
- Geneticist
- Speech-language pathologist
- Occupational therapist
- Physical therapist

Medication

No medications have been approved specifically to treat FASDs. But, several medications can help improve some of the symptoms of FASDs. For example, medication might help manage high energy levels, inability to focus, or depression.

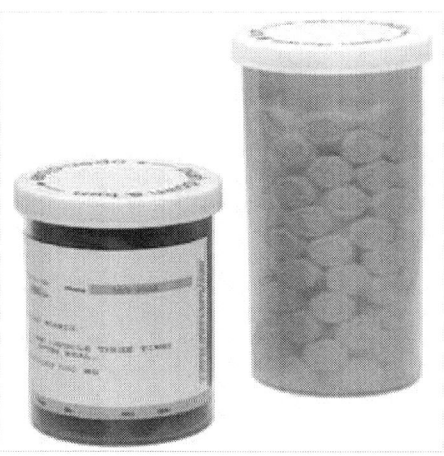

Following are some examples of medications used to treat FASD symptoms:

- **Stimulants.** This type of medication is used to treat symptoms such as hyperactivity, problems paying attention, and poor impulse control, as well as other behavior issues.

- **Antidepressants.** This type of medication is used to treat symptoms such as sad mood, loss of interest, sleep problems, school disruption, negativity, irritability, aggression, and anti-social behaviors.

- **Neuroleptics.** This type of medication is used to treat symptoms such as aggression, anxiety, and certain other behavior problems.

- **Anti-anxiety drugs.** This type of medication is used to treat symptoms of anxiety.

Medications can affect each child differently. One medication might work well for one child, but not for another. To find the right treatment, the doctor might try different medications and doses. It is important to work with your child's doctor to find the treatment plan that works best for your child.

Behavior and Education Therapy

Behavior and education therapy can be an important part of treatment for children with FASDs. Although there are many different types of therapy for children with developmental disabilities, only a few have been scientifically tested specifically for children with FASDs.

Following are behavior and education therapies that have been shown to be effective for some children with FASDs:

- **Friendship training.** Many children with FASDs have a hard time making friends, keeping friends, and socializing with others. Friendship training teaches children with FASDs how to interact with friends, how to enter a group of children already playing, how to arrange and handle in-home play dates, and how to avoid and work out conflicts. A research study found that this type of training could significantly improve children's social skills and reduce problem behaviors.

- **Specialized math tutoring.** A research study found that special teaching methods and tools can help improve math knowledge and skills in children with FASDs.

- **Executive functioning training.** This type of training teaches behavioral awareness and self-control and improves executive functioning skills, such as memory, cause and effect, reasoning, planning, and problem solving.

- **Parent-child interaction therapy.** This type of therapy aims to improve parent-child relationships, create a positive discipline program, and reduce behavior problems in children with FASDs. Parents learn new skills from a coach. A research study found significant decrease in parent distress and child behavior problems.

- **Parenting and behavior management training.** The behavior and learning problems that affect children with FASDs can lead to high levels of stress for the children's parents. This training can improve caregiver comfort, meet family needs, and reduce child problem behaviors.

Parent Training

Children with FASDs might not respond to the usual parenting practices. Parent training has been successful in educating parents about their child's disability and about ways to teach their child many skills and help them cope with their FASD-related symptoms. Parent training can be done in groups or with individual families. Such programs are offered by therapists or in special classes.

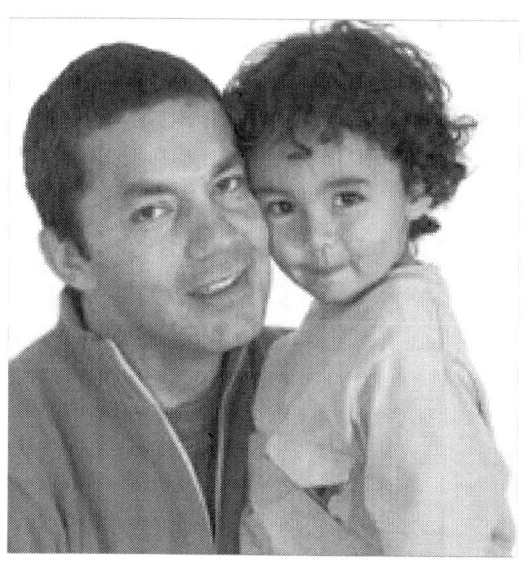

Although each child is unique, the following parenting tips can be helpful:

- Concentrate on your child's strengths and talents
- Accept your child's limitations
- Be consistent with everything (discipline, school, behaviors)
- Use concrete language and examples
- Use stable routines that do not change daily
- Keep it simple
- Be specific-say exactly what you mean
- Structure your child's world to provide a foundation for daily living
- Use visual aids, music, and hands-on activities to help your child learn
- Use positive reinforcement often (praise, incentives)
- Supervise: friends, visits, routines
- Repeat, repeat, repeat

Families might need support from a family counselor or therapist. Parents might also benefit from local support groups, in which parents of children with FASDs can discuss concerns, ask questions, and find encouragement.

Check with one of the following resources to find support in your area:

National and State Resource Directory from the National Organization on Fetal Alcohol Syndrome (NOFAS)

Family Empowerment Network (FEN) - Call 1-800-462-5254 for referrals to services

FASD State Systems of Care from the Substance Abuse and Mental Health Services Administration (SAMHSA) FASD Center for Excellence

Alternative Approaches

With any disability, injury, or medical condition, many untested therapies become known and are promoted by informal networks. These therapies are referred to as alternative treatments. Before starting such a treatment, check it out carefully, and talk to your child's doctor. Your child's doctor will help you weigh the risks and benefits of these therapies.

Some of the alternative treatments used for people with FASDs include:

- Biofeedback
- Auditory training
- Relaxation therapy, visual imagery, and meditation (especially for sleep problems and anxiety)
- Creative art therapy
- Yoga and exercise
- Acupuncture and acupressure
- Massage, Reiki, and energy healing
- Vitamins, herbal supplements, and homeopathy
- Animal-assisted therapy

PREVENTION OF FASD

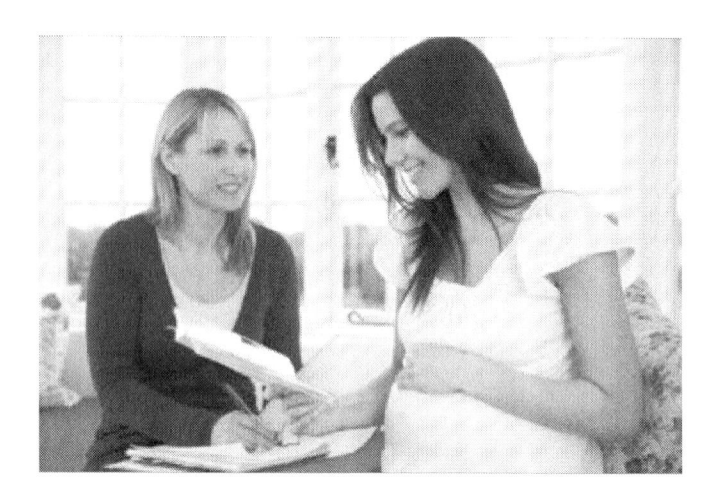

These guidelines can help prevent fetal alcohol syndrome:

- **Don't drink alcohol if you're trying to get pregnant,** because your baby's brain, heart and blood vessels begin to develop in the early weeks of pregnancy, before you may know you're pregnant. If you haven't already stopped drinking, stop as soon as you know you're pregnant or if you even think you might be pregnant. It's never too late to stop drinking during your pregnancy, but the sooner you stop, the better it is for your baby.

- **Continue to avoid alcohol throughout your pregnancy.** Fetal alcohol syndrome is completely preventable in children whose mothers don't drink during pregnancy.

- **Consider giving up alcohol during your childbearing years** if you're sexually active and you're having unprotected sex. Many pregnancies are unplanned, and damage can occur in the earliest weeks of pregnancy.

- **If you have an alcohol problem, get help before you get pregnant.** Get professional help to determine your level of dependence on alcohol and to develop a treatment plan.

In addition, sexually active women who drink heavily should use birth control and control their drinking behaviors.

LIVING WITH FASD

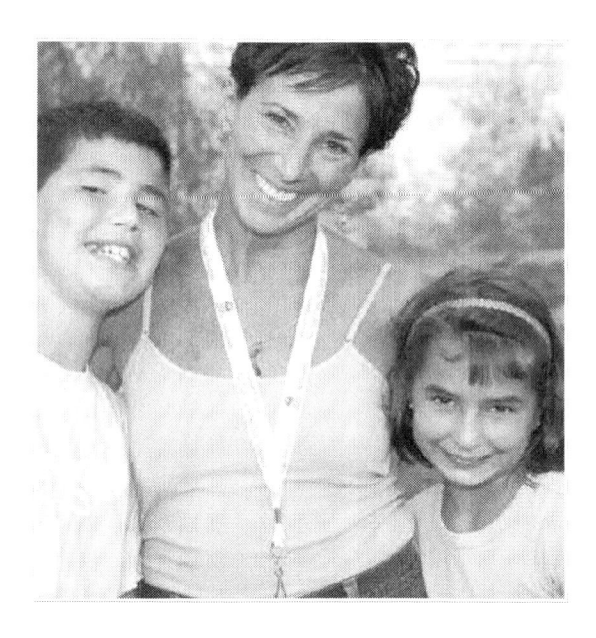

Prenatal exposure to alcohol can result in an almost limitless combination of physical and functional birth defects. While there are specific criteria for diagnosing Fetal Alcohol Syndrome and other disorders under the FASD umbrella, the full range of physical and developmental disabilities for any one affected individual may become evident at irregular times through childhood, adolescence and into adulthood. Preventing the disabilities through early diagnosis and intervention—if possible—and coping with the symptoms or consequences of the disabilities becomes the challenge for families and caregivers.

Described here are practical solutions and brief recommendations for some of the most common challenges, including learning and behavioral problems across the lifespan. Often, more specialized information and resources are needed by families to adequately meet the needs of a loved one with FASD.

FAS/FASD through the Lifespan

FAS/FASD has lifelong implications. There is a broad range of characteristics to watch for at different ages.

- Infants: low birth weight; irritability; sensitivity to light, noises and touch; poor sucking; slow development; poor sleep-wake cycles; increased ear infections.

- Toddlers: poor memory capability, hyperactivity, lack of fear, no sense of boundaries and a need for excessive physical contact.

- Grade-school years: short attention span, poor coordination and difficulty with both fine and gross motor skills.

- Older children: trouble keeping up with school, low self-esteem from recognizing that they are different from their peers.

- Teenagers: poor impulse control, cannot distinguish between public and private behaviors, must be reminded of concepts on a daily basis.

- Adults: need to deal with many daily obstacles, such as affordable and appropriate housing, transportation, employment and money handling.

Strategies for Living

Establish a relationship with a pediatrician and consult him or her with any problems or questions. Here are some other helpful tips.

For Infants:

- Poor sleep-wake cycles/irritability: Play soft music and sing to your baby. Rocking, frequent holding, low lights, automatic swings and wrapping them snugly in a soft blanket also can be helpful.

- Poor weight gain: Consult a nutritionist to develop a food plan or discuss supplement use.

- Chronic ear infections: Speak to a specialist about evaluating your child's hearing and effectively treating infections.

- Delays in rolling over, crawling, walking: See an occupational therapist for assistance. Also help your baby in crawling, grabbing and pulling.

- Speech delays: Consult a speech therapist and purchase tapes or toys that are specifically designed for children with delays. Speak and read aloud expressively to your baby.

Toddlers:

- Continued motor skill delays: Work with an occupational or physical therapist. Use toys that focus on manipulating joints and muscles.

- Distracted easily: Establish a routine and use structure. Simplify rooms in the home and reduce noises or other stimulation.

- Dental problems: Consult a pediatric dentist. Your child may not be able to sit still, so be sure to prepare your child for the exam and allow more time for the appointment.

- Small appetites or sensitivity to food texture: Serve small portions that are lukewarm or cool and have some texture. Allow plenty of time during meals and decrease distractions such as television, radio or multiple conversations.

School age:

- Bedtime: If your child cannot sleep at night, shorten naps or cut them out completely.

- Making and keeping friends: Pair your child with another who is one or two years younger. Provide activities that are short and fun.

- Boundary issues: Create a stable, structured home with clear routines and plenty of repetition.

- Attention problems: Medication may be helpful. Keep the child's environment as simple as possible, and structure time with brief activities.

- Easily frustrated/tantrums: Remove your child from the situation and use calming techniques such as sitting in a rocker, giving a warm bath or playing quiet music.

- Difficulty understanding cause and effect: Repetition, consistency and clear consequences for behavior are important.

Adolescence:

- Anxiety and depression: Medication may be helpful, as well as counseling or encouraging your child to participate in sports, clubs or other structured activities.

- Victimization: Monitor the activities of your child and discuss dealing with strangers.

- Lying, stealing or antisocial behavior: Family counseling is helpful, as well as setting simple and consistent rules with immediate consequences.

Adulthood:

- Housing: Finding appropriate housing for adults affected by FAS/FASD is extremely challenging. Contact your state's department of disabilities to pursue residential funding and get on every waiting list you can find that offers housing options.

- Poor peer or social relations: Enroll your child in classes or social clubs for adults with disabilities.

- Mental health issues: Provide structure, routine and plenty of activities. Investigate medication options and counseling.

- Handling money: Many FAS adults need the family to handle all financial matters.

- Difficulty obtaining or keeping jobs: Investigate trade schools, job training programs or job coaches. Be sure to select jobs that offer structured, routine activities that won't cause overload or stress.

More Tips

Routine:

- Keep your family's routine as consistent as possible.
- If the family's routine or schedule changes, remind your child about changes.

Behavior:

- Learn how to tell when your child is getting frustrated, and help out early.
- Make sure your child understands the rules at home.

- Tell your child about what will happen if he or she has good behavior or bad behavior at home.

- Let your child know when he or she has good behavior.

- Teach self-talk to help your child develop self-control. Use specific, short phrases such as "stop and think."

- Repeat everything you say and give your child many chances to do what you ask.

- Be patient.

- Give directions one step at a time. Wait for your child to do the first step in the directions before telling your child the second step.

- Tell your child before you touch him or her.

- Be sure your child understands your rules, and be firm and consistent with them.

REAL STORIES FROM PEOPLE LIVING WITH FASD

Melissa's Story

This is the story of Melissa's experience with alcohol use during pregnancy and her journey to find the best possible care for her son.

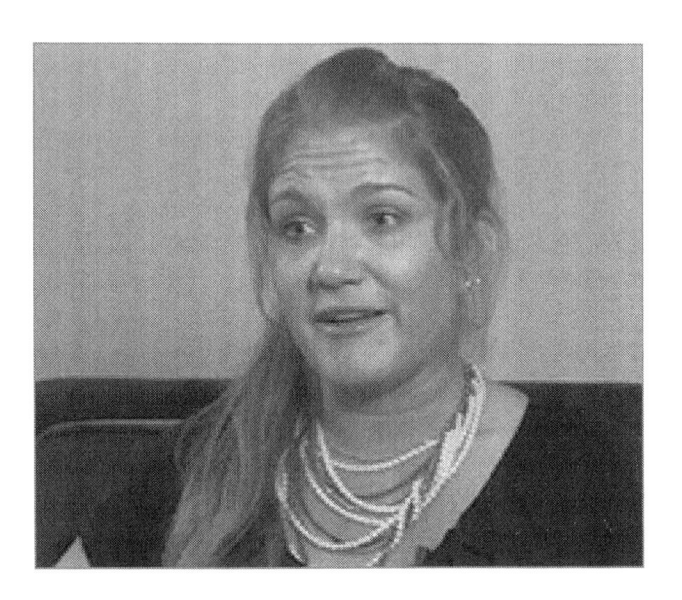

"I drank at the beginning of my pregnancy; before I found out I was pregnant. My doctor told me that it was okay to continue to drink wine during pregnancy. He said I could have a glass of wine at night with dinner. He said it might even help me relax and improve circulation. Not only did I think drinking wine during pregnancy was okay, but I thought that it could be healthy. He never asked me if I had a drinking problem, or how many drinks I have a day, or if I binge drink. There wasn't any dialogue. I really wish that my doctor would have had more dialogue or asked me questions about drinking alcohol during pregnancy.

"When my son was born he looked perfect. He has amazing strengths. He's brilliant and he's an amazing musician. However, as he got older I realized that things just weren't quite right. He doesn't like how clothes feel. He wore the same outfit for almost a year. I finally found a pair of socks that he would wear. Then the company stopped making the sock. That wouldn't be a big deal for most people, but it was a terrifying moment for me. We went through about 25 packages of socks before we found a new brand that he would wear.

"On his first day of kindergarten, the school called me because he had turned over all of the chairs that people weren't sitting in, turned over items in the kitchen area in the classroom, and thrown his shoes at the teacher.

"Most kids will get mad when they have to end play dates or sleepovers. But instead of just getting mad, my son tried to jump out of the car the other day because he had to leave a sleepover.

"When I finally realized what was going on, it was a relief, and it was horrifying, and I felt guilty, and I felt ashamed. But mostly I felt relieved to know what was going on.

"If a pregnant woman said to me, 'I drink a little bit here and there and I was told it was okay,' I would tell her that she wouldn't if she had to live just one day with the way that I feel about myself, knowing how my son has been affected by my choices.

"I am angry that I was given wrong information about drinking during pregnancy. I want to tell as many people as I can about it. **You never know how much alcohol during pregnancy is too much, so why take that chance?"**

Thanks to Melissa and the National Organization on Fetal Alcohol Syndrome (NOFAS) for sharing this story with us.

Frances's Story

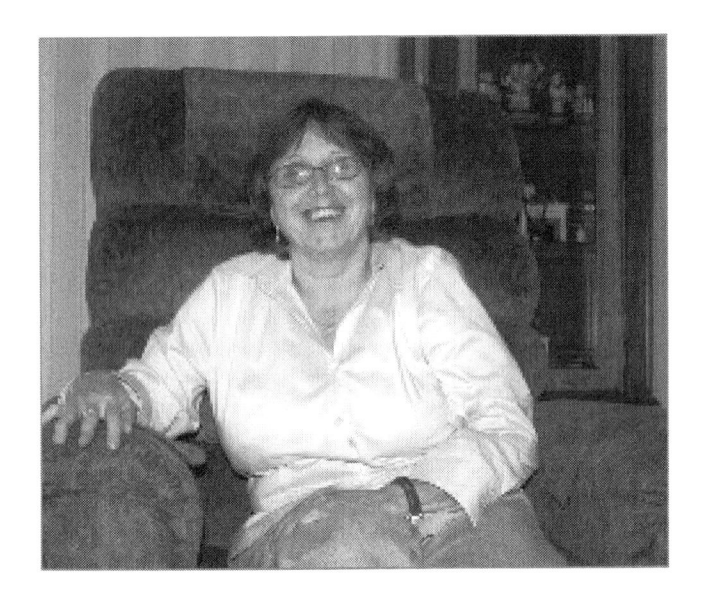

"FASD has affected my life in many ways. I was born six weeks early and weighed three pounds, eleven ounces. As a child, I never knew what it was but it was hard for me to make friends and I found myself feeling afraid of others. School was very hard for me, especially math and English. I couldn't comprehend them. I completed high school and tried college, but it didn't go well. Then I got a job.

"Working was hard. I didn't know what I wanted to do and I went from job to job. I couldn't hold on to a job. It was hard for me because I developed anxiety, depression and an eating disorder. I still deal with that today. I see a therapist often and take medication. It's still a struggle.

"I do a lot of writing to express my feelings. It helps me. I also watch people very carefully to learn how to do certain things. I tend to read everything twice to comprehend what I am reading. For my anxiety, I avoid loud and crowded places. I always surround myself with people that I feel comfortable and safe with.

"I got involved with an organization called Al-Anon because I grew up in an alcoholic family. I do share my FASD story at the Al-Anon meetings. **I always tell myself if there is one young woman who is thinking about having a child and who is drinking, if I share my story and that one person hears me, it's worth it.**

"I want people to know that there is hope. I keep telling myself, if I can survive, others can too. FASD comes with a lot of shame and challenges. I always tell people to stop and think before taking that drink. Pregnant women should remember that they are not drinking alone."

Thanks to Frances and the National Organization on Fetal Alcohol Syndrome (NOFAS) for sharing this personal story.

RESEARCH ON FASD

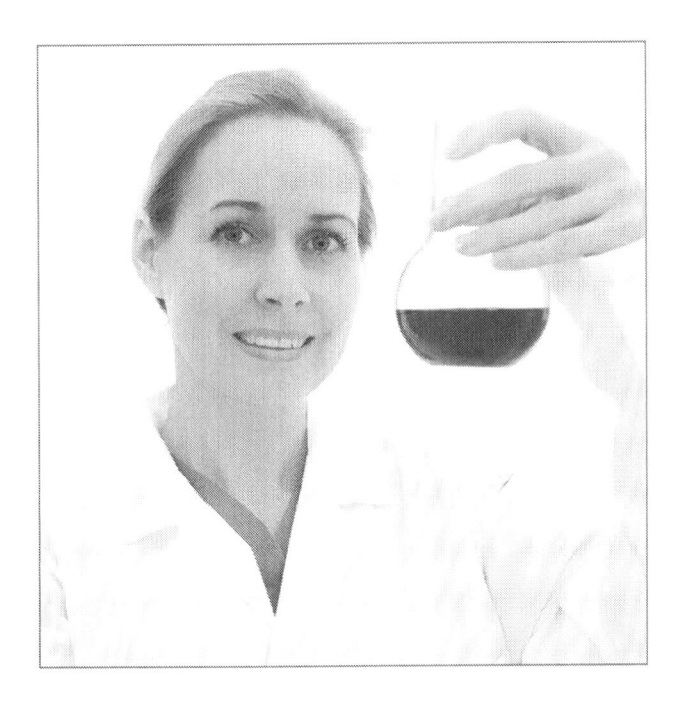

The National Institute on Alcohol Abuse and Alcoholism—part of the National Institutes of Health, the Nation's medical research agency—has a large research program on fetal alcohol spectrum disorders (FASD) that sponsors projects on prevention, treatment of women with alcohol use disorders, improving diagnosis of FASD, increasing understanding of the effects of alcohol on the unborn child, and developing effective interventions to mitigate the health effects on those prenatally exposed to alcohol.

NIAAA's FASD Grant Portfolio: Annually, NIAAA expends 8-9% of its extramural research and training budget, or roughly $30 million, toward its portfolio of FASD-related grants. This portfolio is comprised of approximately 100 grants, including research program grants, cooperative agreements, training grants, center grants, fellowships, and career development awards, that collectively address FASD prevention, diagnosis, treatment, and etiology. In addition, NIAAA funds a conference grant that supports the annual meeting of the FASD Study Group.

The Collaborative Initiative on Fetal Alcohol Spectrum Disorders (CIFASD) is a multidisciplinary consortium of domestic and international projects established by NIAAA in 2003 to address the prevention of Fetal Alcohol Spectrum Disorders (FASD), the diagnosis of the full range of birth defects associated with prenatal alcohol exposure, and ameliorative interventions for affected individuals. CIFASD aims to accelerate the translation of key research findings by fostering collaboration and coordinating clinical, basic, and translational research.

The Prenatal Alcohol and Sudden Infant Death Syndrome and Stillbirth (PASS) Network is an international consortium investigating the role of prenatal alcohol exposure in the risk for Sudden Infant Death Syndrome (SIDS), stillbirth, and FASD. The PASS Network is conducting community-based investigations known as the Safe Passage Study in high-risk communities of the Northern Plains of the United States and the Western Cape of South Africa. This prospective study plans to enroll approximately 12,000 pregnant women and follow the development of their offspring through pregnancy and the infants' first year of life. NIAAA funds the PASS Network in partnership with the Eunice Kennedy Shriver National Institute of Child Health and Human Development (NICHD) and the National Institute on Deafness and Other Communication Disorders (NIDCD).

The Collaboration on FASD Prevalence (CoFASP) research consortium, comprised of research teams led by Drs. Christina Chambers and Phil May, seeks to establish the prevalence of FASD among school-aged children in several U.S. communities, located in California, North Carolina, and the Northern Plains, using active case ascertainment methodology. In addition to establishing a more precise and representative prevalence estimate through standardized diagnostic criteria for FASD, NIAAA's goal for this initiative is to establish a publically available database to facilitate future FASD research.

Understanding and Improving Health Messages about Alcohol and Pregnancy

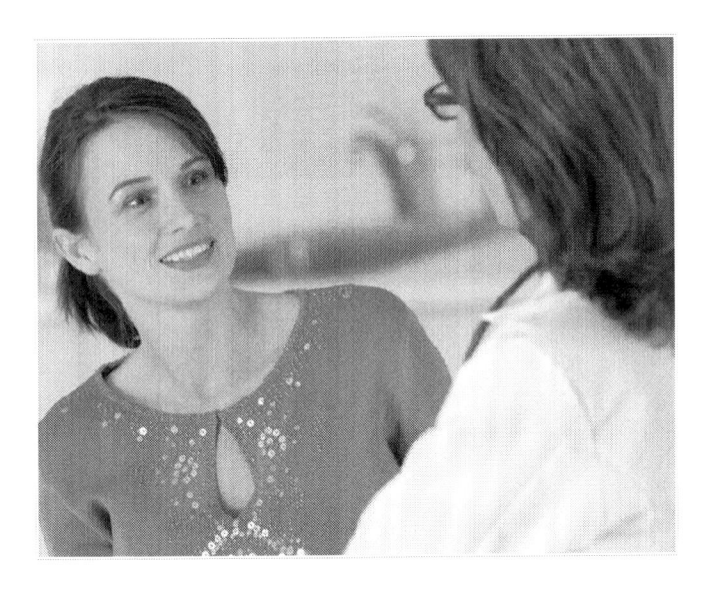

The American Journal of Health Education published a study looking at women's knowledge and beliefs about alcohol use and its risks during pregnancy, the role others play in influencing women's behaviors, and women's sources of health information to understand this issue. The study also provides suggestions based on these findings for health educators and communicators to consider when developing messages and materials for women about alcohol use and pregnancy.

Main Findings from this Study

- While women recognized the risks and consequences of drinking alcohol during pregnancy, many still held common **misconceptions**.
    - Some women reported that certain kinds of alcohol are okay to drink during pregnancy and that drinking

in the third trimester (last 3 months of pregnancy) did not harm the developing baby.

- o Others thought that drinking small amounts of alcohol during pregnancy was acceptable and some said that their health care providers agreed that it was okay to drink small amounts.

- o Some women continued to drink alcohol during pregnancy or said that they intended to continue drinking until it was confirmed that they were pregnant.

- A woman's partner, family, and friends influence her decisions whether or not to drink alcohol during pregnancy. Health care providers and the Internet act as important sources of health information for women, but do not always provide consistent information about the risks of alcohol use during pregnancy.

- Education and awareness among women and health care professionals about the risks of alcohol use during pregnancy continue to be important to prevent alcohol-exposed pregnancies and fetal alcohol spectrum disorders. Considerations for messaging and educational materials related to alcohol use and pregnancy include providing clear and consistent messaging (especially from health care professionals), focusing on social support strategies, and utilizing electronic media.

About this Study

Basics about Fetal Alcohol Spectrum Disorders

- Alcohol use during pregnancy can cause birth defects and developmental disabilities collectively known as fetal alcohol spectrum disorders (FASDs). It can also cause other pregnancy problems, such as miscarriage, stillbirth, and prematurity.

- There is *no* guaranteed safe level of alcohol use at any time during pregnancy or when trying to get pregnant. All kinds of alcohol should be avoided, including red or white wine, beer, and liquor.

- Alcohol can cause problems for a developing baby throughout pregnancy, including before a woman knows she is pregnant.

- Fetal alcohol spectrum disorders are completely preventable if a woman doesn't drink during pregnancy. Why take the risk?

Researchers conducted 20 focus groups with 149 women of reproductive age segmented by age, pregnancy status, and race/ethnicity. Data were coded and analyzed across several categories (for example, knowledge and beliefs, misconceptions, social influences, information sources).

The Consequences of Prenatal Alcohol Exposure

In the early 1990s, NIAAA funded seminal research by Dr. Edward Riley and colleagues, which used noninvasive imaging to show that multiple areas of the central nervous system are adversely affected by prenatal alcohol exposure. Structural imaging studies confirmed reductions in the volume of overall brain size, with disproportionate reductions in basal ganglia and the anterior vermis of the cerebellum. Additional studies have shown alterations in brain shape, changes in cortical thickness, reduced size, and altered shape of the corpus callosum, as well as alterations in the hippocampus.

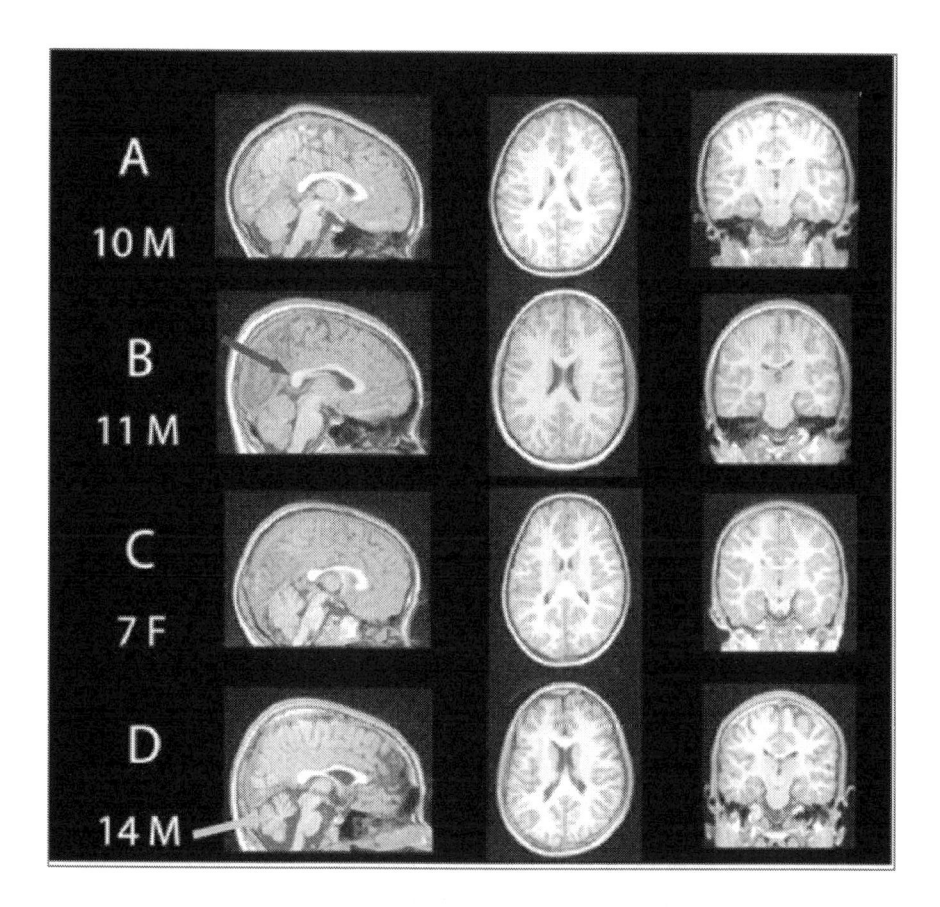

Magnetic Resonance Imaging (MRI) scans of four children: (A) shows a typically developing 10-year-old boy who has not been exposed to alcohol (B) features an 11-year-old boy with partial fetal alcohol syndrome (pFAS) (C) shows a 7-year-old girl with FAS, and (D) shows a 14-year-old boy with FAS. Notice the variability in brain structures among the individuals with fetal alcohol syndrome disorders, including alcohol-related changes in areas such as the corpus callosum (red arrow) and cerebellum (yellow arrow). SOURCE: Sowell, E.; Nunez, S.; Roussotte, F. Structural and functional brain abnormalities in fetal alcohol spectrum disorders, *Alcohol Research & Health*, in press.

Since those early studies, a variety of imaging techniques have been used, including diffusion tensor imaging, magnetic resonance spectroscopy, functional magnetic resonance imaging, positron emission tomography, and single-photon emission computed tomography. These studies show that prenatal alcohol exposure disrupts development of both gray and white matter and further illustrate alcohol-related alterations in cerebral blood flow, neurotransmitters, and neuronal activity, even when there are no obvious structural changes. Importantly, it was discovered that individuals exposed to alcohol prenatally could suffer from brain anomalies and dysfunction without exhibiting distinct facial dysmorphology, a finding with significant implications for the identification of children with FASD. More recently, prenatal and neonatal ultrasound are being used to help identify brain anomalies early in development, which may be key for early intervention. NIAAA also is now supporting similar brain-imaging techniques with animal models, in which alcohol exposure parameters can be controlled.

The neuropathology associated with FASD leads to a range of behavioral effects. Early studies demonstrated general impairments in intelligence (although there is quite a range of IQ scores among individuals exposed to alcohol prenatally), impaired reflex development, deficits in motor coordination, and hyperactivity. More recent studies suggest that deficits in attention, learning and memory, emotional dysregulation, and executive functioning are core deficits, likely reflecting the dysfunction of the frontal lobe. These behavioral domains also are disrupted with animal models of FASD. Moreover, prenatal alcohol-induced alterations in cognitive functioning and stress responses may contribute to secondary disabilities, including psychiatric comorbidities and vulnerability to addiction. One of the challenges is to determine if there is a pattern of neuropathology and behavioral expression that is unique to prenatal alcohol exposure and therefore useful for diagnosis, as described below.

Prenatal alcohol also leads to physical and physiological changes that are not part of an FAS diagnosis, including alterations in skeletal and organ formation as well as immune function. Prenatal alcohol exposure also may contribute to other disorders. For example, it may disrupt the development of brain structures that contribute to sudden infant death syndrome. NIAAA is addressing this issue jointly with the National Institute on Child Health and

Human Development via a consortium. When considering that 40 years ago it was not commonly recognized that alcohol was a teratogen, remarkable strides have been made in understanding the range of ethanol's adverse effects on the developing embryo and fetus.

Dysregulation of microRNA Expression and Function Contributes to the Etiology of Fetal Alcohol Spectrum Disorders

MicroRNAs (miRNAs) are members of a vast, evolutionarily ancient, but poorly understood class of regulatory RNA molecules, termed non–protein-coding RNAs (ncRNAs). This means that in contrast to RNA molecules generated during gene expression (i.e., messenger RNA [mRNA] molecules), they are not used as templates for the synthesis of proteins. ncRNAs are encoded within the genomes of both eukaryotic and prokaryotic organisms and represent a novel layer of cell regulation and function that rivals the diversity and function of protein-coding mRNAs.

In recent years, researchers have investigated whether, and how, miRNAs interact with beverage alcohol (i.e., ethanol) and/or mediate its effects. Initial studies explored the ethanol–miRNA interactions in fetal neural stem cells. Since then, increasing evidence has indicated that miRNAs play a role in the etiology of alcoholism and potentially alcohol withdrawal, as well as in ethanol's effects on brain development, brain damage associated with adult alcoholism, and liver damage (i.e., hepatotoxicity). Other drugs of abuse such as nicotine are also known to influence miRNA expression; furthermore, ethanol and nicotine collaborate to regulate the expression of miRNAs in neural tissues. These data collectively suggest that miRNAs are an important, but as yet poorly understood, component of alcoholism and ethanol-associated toxicology and damage to the developing fetus (i.e., teratology). This review specifically focuses on the association between miRNAs and the developmental effects of ethanol exposure, examining both the current data and future potential for research in this field of ncRNA biology to promote a coherent understanding of teratology associated with alcohol exposure.

Focus on miRNAs

miRNAs are a class of ncRNAs that posttranscriptionally regulate the expression of protein-coding genes. When protein-coding genes are expressed (i.e., the encoded protein is produced), first an mRNA copy of the corresponding DNA sequence is generated in a process called transcription. This mRNA molecule consists of three parts: a noncoding start region (i.e., the 5'-end), the sequence actually containing the information for the encoded protein (i.e., the open reading frame), and a noncoding tail region (i.e., the 3'-end). miRNAs mainly act by binding to the 3'-untranslated region of their mRNA targets, although that is not the only function attributable to these molecules. Many microRNAs are evolutionarily conserved across species. They initially were discovered in the roundworm *Caenorhabditis elegans*, but since then they also have been found in plants, invertebrates, mammals, and humans. miRNAs play crucial roles in development, stem-cell self-renewal, programmed cell death (i.e., apoptosis), and cell-cycle regulation but also feature prominently in human disease, including cancers and neurodegenerative and metabolic diseases. miRNAs are abundant in the central nervous system (CNS), and brain miRNAs are crucial for regulating nerve cell generation (i.e., neurogenesis); neuronal degeneration; and maintaining normal neuronal functions associated with memory formation, neuronal differentiation, and synaptic plasticity.

miRNA Biogenesis

miRNAs are encoded within the genome either as independent genes or in gene clusters; however, they also can be encoded within introns of protein-coding genes, or even within introns and exons of another type of ncRNA called long intergenic non-(protein)-coding RNAs (lincRNAs). The generation of mature miRNAs from these coding sequences is a multistep process, as follows:

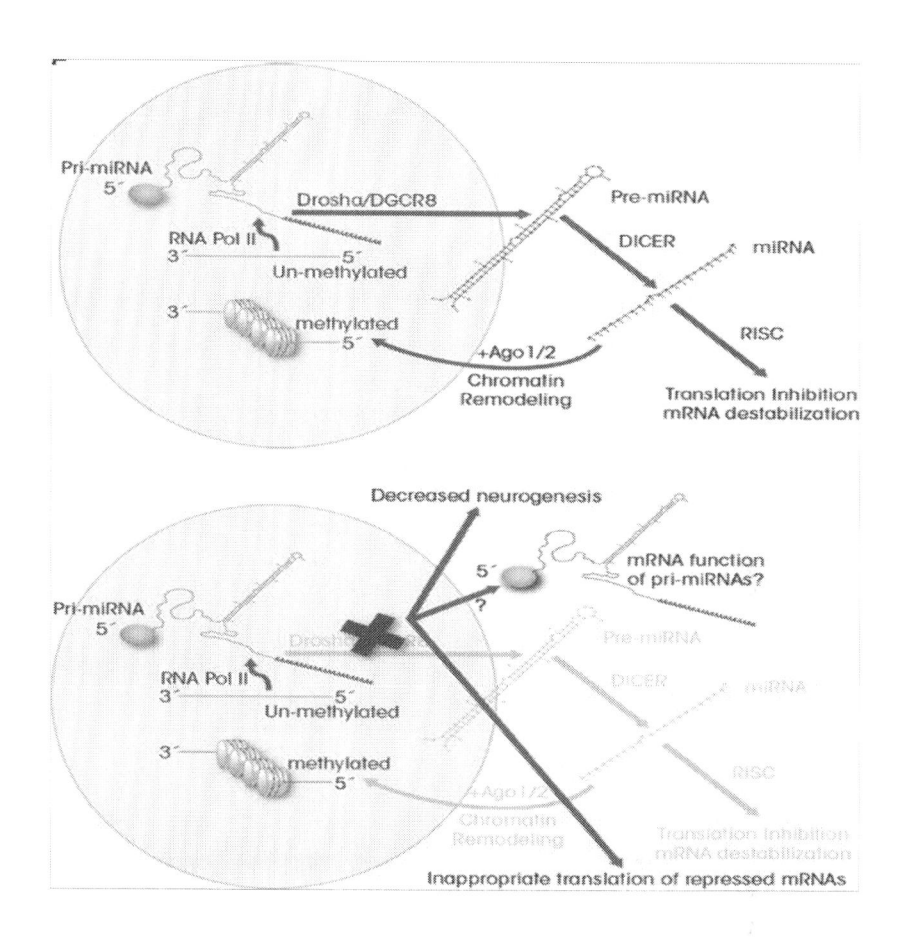

- A normal transcription process, which is mediated by an enzyme called RNA-polymerase II, generates a longer primary transcript termed pri-miRNA. Like mRNA, the pri-miRNA transcripts can have certain modifications at their ends (i.e., a "cap" at the 5′-end and multiple adenosine units [i.e., a poly-A tail] at the 3′-end) and can be spliced. Furthermore, the pri-miRNAs typically are folded into a double-stranded, hairpin–loop structure several hundred base pairs in length.

- Most pri-miRNA transcripts are processed within the nucleus by a protein complex called the DiGeorge syndrome critical region-8 (Drosha/DGCR8) "microprocessor" complex to generate stem-loop structures termed pre-miRNAs that are approximately 70 nucleotides in length.

- The pre-miRNAs are moved from the nucleus to the cytoplasm by a chaperone protein called exportin-5.

- Within the cytoplasm, a protein complex known as Dicer enzyme further processes pre-miRNAs into mature double-stranded miRNA molecules. This process, and thus miRNA formation in general, is crucial for embryonic development because mutations in the Dicer proteins, which are exclusively part of the miRNA processing machinery, cause death of the embryo.

- Once the Dicer complex is cut off to release the mature miRNA, one strand of the double-stranded molecule, termed the guide strand miRNA, preferentially attaches to another protein complex called RNA-induced silencing complex (RISC). This results in a microribonucleoprotein (miRNP) complex that can either destabilize mRNA transcripts or repress the next step of gene expression in protein-coding genes (i.e., translation). The second, complementary strand, known as passenger strand or miRNA* has been thought to be quickly degraded. However, as discussed later in this article, recent studies indicate that passenger-strand miRNAs can be retained by cells and exhibit independent biological functions.

Model for the activity of the two strands of the processed pre-miRNA molecules (i.e., the guide strand [miRNA] and passenger strand [miRNA*]). Dicer processing of pre-miRNAs typically results in the formation of a guide stand miRNA that binds to the RNA-induced.

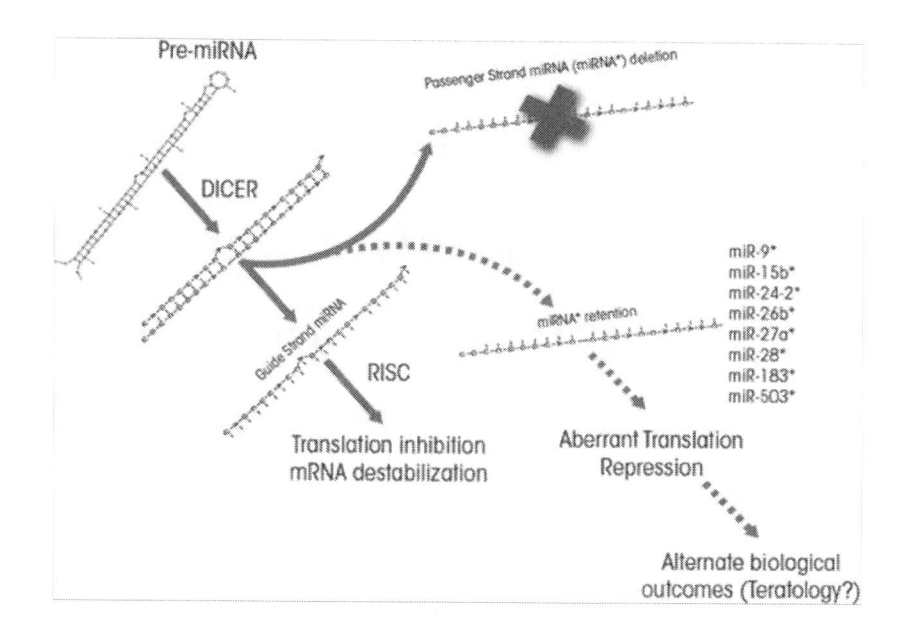

- Finally, the mature miRNA can be degraded by an enzyme called 5′-3′ exoribonuclease (XRN2).

Models for standard (i.e., canonical) and disturbed (i.e., noncanonical) modes of miRNA biogenesis and function. miRNAs often are generated (i.e., transcribed) from miRNA genes, as long mRNA-like transcripts, with a "cap" at the start.

Role of miRNAs in Ethanol's Teratologic Effects

In 2007, Sathyan and colleagues (2007) showed for the first time that miRNAs could mediate the effects of ethanol or indeed other teratogens. Using isolated tissue from the nervous system (i.e., neuroepithelium) of second-trimester fetuses, the investigators demonstrated that ethanol suppressed the expression of four miRNAs—miR-9, miR-21, miR-153, and miR-335—in fetal neural stem cells (NSCs) and neural progenitor cells (NPCs). The simultaneous suppression of miR-21 and miR-335 accounted for earlier observations that ethanol-exposed NSCs/NPCs are resistant to apoptosis, whereas the suppression of miR-335 explained the increase in NSC/NPC proliferation. Three of the four suppressed miRNAs target the mRNAs for two proteins called Jagged-1 and ELAVL2/HuB; accordingly, by suppressing the miRNAs, ethanol induced the expression of both target mRNAs. ELAVL2/HuB overexpression promotes neuronal differentiation, and Jagged-1–induced proliferation establishes neuronal identity. These data collectively suggest that by interfering with miRNA function, ethanol may deplete the fetal pool of NSCs/NPCs and promote premature neuronal differentiation. More recently, Tal and colleagues (2012), using a zebrafish model, also showed that ethanol exposure during embryonic development suppressed the expression of miR-9 and miR-153. Importantly, these investigators demonstrated both behavioral and anatomical consequences of miRNA depletion. In particular, miR-153 depletion resulted in significantly increased locomotor activity in juvenile zebrafish, reminiscent of increased hyperactivity observed in children with FASD.

Other developmental ethanol exposure models also have indicated that ethanol alters the expression of several miRNAs. For example, Wang and colleagues (2009) showed that ethanol exposure during a period bracketing the end of the first trimester to the middle of the second trimester resulted in altered miRNA expression in brain tissue sampled near the end of the second trimester. In that study, ethanol induced a significant increase in the expression of two miRNAs (i.e., miR-10a and miR-10b), resulting in down-regulated expression of a protein called Hoxa1 in fetal brains. Other analyses had indicated that loss of Hoxa1 function (e.g., from familial Hoxa1 mutations) is associated with a variety of cranial defects and mental retardation. This suggests that by suppressing translation of Hoxa1 and related genes, ethanol-mediated induction of miR10a/b may lead to similar defects.

Although the miRNAs identified by Wang and colleagues (2009) do not overlap with those identified by Sathyan and colleagues (2007) in NSCs/NPCs, miR-10a/b upregulation may have similar consequences for premature NSC differentiation. For example, miR-10a/b promotes the differentiation of cells from a type of nerve cell tumor (i.e., neuroblastoma cells) by suppressing translation of a protein called nuclear receptor corepressor-2 (NCOR2). This effect is similar to the induction of Elavl2/HuB and Jagged-1.

Finally, Guo and colleagues (2011) assessed the effects of chronic intermittent ethanol exposure on cultured neuronal cells obtained from mouse cerebral cortex at gestational day 15, which is equivalent to the middle of the second trimester. The investigators found that ethanol induced several miRNAs in these cells. Interestingly, a prolonged period of withdrawal following the ethanol exposure resulted in a more than fourfold increase in the number of significantly regulated miRNAs, suggesting that withdrawal itself also may have a significant damaging effect on neuronal maturation in the developing fetal brain. Although these data were obtained from a cell-culture model, the implications of maternal binge drinking–withdrawal cycles on fetal miRNAs and their control over neural differentiation need further investigation.

Effects of Coexposure to Ethanol and Other Drugs on miRNA Levels

Pregnant women who abuse ethanol also are likely to coabuse other drugs, such as nicotine. These other drugs also can affect miRNA levels. For example, Huang and colleagues (2009) demonstrated that nicotine induced expression of miR140* in a developmental model using the rat PC12 cell line. These effects may enhance or oppose those of ethanol. Thus, a recent study showed that ethanol and nicotine behaved as functional antagonists—that is, miRNAs that were suppressed by ethanol in fetal NSCs/NPCs were induced by nicotine exposure. Moreover, nicotine prevented the ethanol-mediated decrease in these miRNAs; this effect was pharmacologically mediated by a certain type of nicotine receptor (i.e., the nicotinic acetylcholine receptor). There is little generalized evidence as yet that drugs of abuse interact at the level of miRNAs to regulate cell function. Nevertheless these findings suggested that such an interaction is a real possibility, and the consequences for the teratologic effects of the drugs are likely to be significant.

Teratogenic Implications of Altered miRNA Biogenesis, Cellular Localization, and Function

The data cited above show that ethanol alters the expression of several miRNAs at different developmental stages and that these alterations have consequences for fetal neural development and behavior. miRNA dysregulation is likely to influence teratogenesis by destabilizing the mRNAs of individual genes or gene networks. However, emerging evidence indicates that miRNA function also can be altered at several stages in the miRNA biogenesis pathway. Although to date such alterations are poorly understood, they may have important implications for teratology. The following represent four intriguing possibilities.

First, the presence of a 5' cap and a 3'-polyA tail indicates that primary miRNA transcripts may have characteristics and function like regular mRNAs, and indeed evidence has been found for such a role. Although the conditions that permit the appearance of mRNA-like functionality are unclear, it is likely that interference with Dicer/DGCR8, which is essential for miRNA processing, can lead to the emergence of alternate functionality associated with pri-miRNA transcripts. In this context, it is interesting to note that disruption of the DGCR8 locus is associated with mental retardation and that DGCR8 deletion interferes with the maturation of embryonic stem cells, causing them to aberrantly retain their ability to differentiate into different cell types (i.e., their pluripotency) while initiating differentiation. In this instance, the biology of stem cells seems to be intimately linked with the development of normal brain function.

Second, until recently, the complementary miRNA* strands were thought to be quickly degraded following Dicer cleavage of the double-stranded pre-miRNA molecule. However, recent evidence shows that these passenger strands also can be functional, acting on their own binding sites and regulating expression of their own sets of targets. Thus, both strands of a premiRNA can be functional, each with a specific set of targets. The ratio of functional guide versus passenger strand miRNAs is regulated by an as-yet-unknown biology. Guo and colleagues (2011) identified several ethanol-sensitive miRNA* species that mainly were induced following ethanol exposure. Furthermore, other drugs of abuse, such as nicotine, also have been shown to induce the expression of a miRNA* (i.e., miR140*). Alterations in the miRNA-to-miRNA*s ratio are likely to yield alternate biological outcomes that are particularly relevant to teratogenesis, as has been demonstrated in an analysis of the established ethanol-sensitive miRNA, miR-9. Tal and colleagues (2012) showed in their developmental zebrafish model that in addition to decreasing miR-9 (which now is also called miR-9-5p), ethanol produced a more modest decrease in the expression of miR-9* (now called miR-9-3p). The ratio of miR-9 to miR-9* is important for development and teratogenesis because these two miRNAs work together to regulate two molecules controlling neuronal differentiation. Thus, miR-9 levels influence the levels of a neuronal differentiation inhibitor called RE1 silencing transcription factor/neuron-restrictive silencer factor (REST), whereas miR-9* regulates its cofactor, coREST. Therefore, the simultaneous suppression of miR-9 and miR-9* may be expected to result in derepression of the REST/coREST complex and, consequently, inhibition of neuronal differentiation. On the other hand, preferential suppression of either miR-9 or miR-9* would be predicted to alter the ratio of REST to coREST, which has important and complex consequences for neural stem-cell renewal and altered lineage specification. Clearly, the involvement of passenger-strand miRNA biology in teratogenesis needs further investigation.

Third, in humans, about 6 percent of mature miRNAs undergo editing by the enzyme adenosine deaminase, resulting in alterations in either miRNA processing or miRNA efficiency. Furthermore, evidence suggests that edited miRNAs may exhibit different target specificity compared with their nonedited counterparts. miRNA editing increases during brain development and may permit the emergence of new biological functions (e.g., a novel translational control of the development of nerve cell extensions [i.e., dendritogenesis]). These data collectively suggest that the role of miRNA editing in ethanol teratology warrants further exploration.

Finally, emerging evidence indicates that some mature miRNAs are transported back to the nucleus, where they mediate the formation of heterochromatin. This observation suggests that miRNAs can directly influence the epigenetic landscape. Ethanol also alters the epigenetic landscape in differentiating fetal NSCs, and the contributory role of nuclear miRNAs to this process is unknown. All of these modifications to miRNA biology represent novel and uninvestigated layers of regulatory processes that may have important consequences for cell and tissue differentiation and, consequently, teratogenesis.

Implications for the Management of FASD

Despite strong evidence that maternal alcohol consumption during pregnancy leads to harmful effects on the fetus, a significant number of women continue to report drinking even into the third trimester of pregnancy. Therefore, early detection and management of fetal alcohol exposure remains an urgent public health concern, as does the development of approaches to ameliorate or prevent ethanol's detrimental effects. The identification of miRNAs as ethanol targets presents one hope for the development of novel therapeutic programs. miRNAs have coevolved with their mRNA targets to orchestrate development. It is possible that miRNA-like drugs may be used to mitigate the effects of fetal ethanol exposure on the development of specific organs. The challenge will be to identify tissue-specific miRNAs that can be used to reprogram development. In this context, miRNAs such as miR-9 make intriguing therapeutic targets because they are fairly specific to neuronal cells. Evidence that ethanol-sensitive miRNAs also are sensitive to nicotine suggests a promising and alternative, pharmacological approach to reprogramming fetal development following maternal ethanol exposure. Recent evidence suggests that pharmacologic approaches can indeed be used successfully in human populations, for example, to normalize cellular miRNA levels in neurological diseases such as multiple sclerosis. Such an approach therefore may be similarly efficacious with FASD. Finally, Guo and colleagues (2011) have implicated DNA methylation as a mechanism for miRNA regulation, and Wang and colleagues (2009) demonstrated that folic acid administration could reverse ethanol's effects on miRNAs. These data suggest that nutritional supplementation programs also may be an effective means towards ameliorating the effects of miRNA dysregulation. Research into miRNA involvement in fetal alcohol teratology is in its infancy. However, this research has significant potential for both uncovering principles underlying alcohol's detrimental consequences and for developing novel strategies for the management of fetal alcohol effects.

DISTINGUISHING BETWEEN ADHD & FASD IN CHILDREN

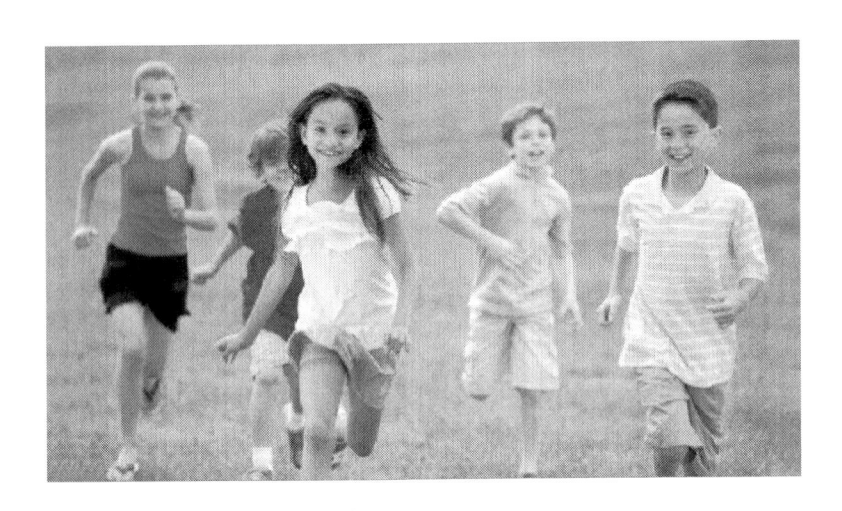

Disruptive, hyperactive, and impulsive behaviors are highly prevalent in individuals with fetal alcohol spectrum disorders (FASD). In this paper we discuss the relationship between attention deficit hyperactivity disorder (ADHD) and FASD. Firstly, we define ADHD and FASD and review the epidemiology of these conditions. Then we discuss the rationale for distinguishing between ADHD with and without FASD and review the evidence regarding the relationship between ADHD and FASD. Finally, we discuss the approach to diagnosis and management of ADHD in individuals with FASD.

Attention Deficit Hyperactivity Disorder

ADHD may be thought of as a group of conditions with similar behavioral symptoms consequent to different etiologies. ADHD is defined as a persistent pattern of behavior including hyperactivity and impulsivity, and/or inattention that is more severe and frequent than is usually seen in an individual at the same stage of development. The Diagnostic and Statistical Manual of Mental Disorders, 4th Edition (DSM-IV) defines three subtypes, ie, a combined type which includes symptoms of inattention and hyperactivity or impulsivity, a predominantly inattentive type, in which hyperactive and impulsive symptoms are minor, and a predominantly hyperactive-impulsive type, in which inattentive symptoms are minor. The subtypes may be discontinued in DSM-5. The mean intelligence quotient (IQ) score and IQ distribution in the ADHD population are similar to that in the general population. ADHD is a neurobiologic disorder with genetic and environmental origins. Family, adoption, and twin studies demonstrate a strong genetic contribution to ADHD, which involves polymorphisms in a number of genes, such as those which code for dopamine transporters. Environmental risk factors for ADHD include antenatal exposure to toxins, such as alcohol and tobacco, prematurity, adverse childhood experiences, childhood illness, head trauma, and exposure to environmental toxins. The heterogeneity of ADHD may be explained partially by the varying contribution of genes and environmental factors for individual children. ADHD is reported in all ethnic groups and social classes. The prevalence of ADHD in children in the general population ranges from 5% to 11%.

Fetal Alcohol Spectrum Disorders

Fetal alcohol syndrome (FAS) was first described in 1973, but descriptions of the effects of alcohol exposure during pregnancy date back to ancient history. FASD is a nondiagnostic umbrella term for the possible childhood outcomes of prenatal alcohol exposure. FASD includes FAS, partial FAS, alcohol-related neurodevelopmental disorder (ARND), and alcohol-related birth defects. Individuals with FAS have specific facial features (including short palpebral fissures, flat philtrum, and thin upper lip), impaired prenatal and/or postnatal growth, and structural or functional problems of the central nervous system. If all of these features are present and differential diagnoses are excluded, the diagnosis of FAS can be made even if alcohol exposure during pregnancy is not confirmed. Individuals with partial FAS have most, but not all, the features of FAS. Individuals with ARND have a complex pattern of behavioral and/or neurologic impairment without the physical features of FAS. Fetal alcohol effects (FAE) is an obsolete term previously used to describe individuals with incomplete features of FAS. The facial features of FAS occur with fetal alcohol exposure early in the first trimester, but neuropsychologic deficits may occur independent of the physical features of FAS. In FAS, IQ scores are reported to range from 20 to 120 with an average IQ score between 68 and 72. Individuals with ARND have a slightly higher IQ than individuals with FAS. Internationally, several diagnostic approaches to FASD have been proposed. Although the diagnostic criteria and terminology used differ only slightly, the use of different approaches is confusing and makes comparison of study results difficult. The estimated prevalence of FAS is 0.5–2.0 per 1000 births, although a prevalence of up to 68 per 1000 has been reported in some high-risk communities. The prevalence of the other FASD diagnoses is not well defined, but it is estimated that FASD affects 1% of all births in the US.

Many studies have focused on defining the behavioral phenotype of FASD to assist diagnosis and intervention. Individuals with FASD frequently display deficits in executive functioning, memory, attention, visual-spatial abilities, planning, cognitive flexibility, processing speed, inhibition and inhibition/switching, deductive reasoning and verbal abstract thinking, problem solving, verbal and spatial concept formation, phonemic switching and phonologic working memory, and motor skills. Executive function deficits are present in individuals with FASD whether or not they have FAS. Older children with FASD are more impaired than younger children on verbal processing tasks. These deficits may contribute to lower IQ scores, poor academic achievement, and learning problems. Long-term studies show that adolescents and young adults with FASD have high rates of secondary disabilities including mental health problems (90%), inappropriate sexual behavior (49%), disrupted school education (60%), and trouble with the law (60%). More than one third experience drug and alcohol problems. These secondary disabilities may arise from the neurobehavioral deficits caused by prenatal alcohol exposure, with exacerbation or amelioration by environmental factors.

Attention and Hyperactivity Problems in FASD

Children with FASD are often described as hyperactive, distractible, and impulsive, with short attention spans. ADHD is the most commonly reported mental health diagnosis in individuals with prenatal alcohol exposure. The prevalence of ADHD (diagnosed according to DSM-IV criteria) in children with heavy prenatal alcohol exposure is between 49.4% and 94%. Unfortunately, prevalence studies have included children with heavy prenatal alcohol exposure (variously defined), with and without a diagnosis of FASD, hence the wide prevalence range. However, the prevalence of ADHD in cohorts with FASD is consistently much higher than that in the general population. The proportion of children with a diagnosis of ADHD who also have FASD is not known and will be influenced by underdiagnosis of FASD. Underdiagnosis occurs due to a variety of factors, including health professionals' reluctance to ask about alcohol exposure in pregnancy or to make a diagnosis due to lack of knowledge or fear of stigmatizing the child. The proportion of children with FAS diagnosed with ADHD increases with the level of alcohol exposure. Attention deficit in individuals with FASD is independent of IQ and persists into adolescence and adulthood. Inattention symptoms are more commonly reported in children with FASD who meet DSM-IV criteria for ADHD, than in children with ADHD who do not have FASD.

Rationale for Distinguishing between ADHD and FASD

The prognosis and treatment responses for children with ADHD and FASD differ to those of children with ADHD alone. Children with FASD often present with early onset ADHD with predominant inattentive symptoms. They are at high risk of secondary disabilities, which can be ameliorated by early diagnosis of FASD and management of its symptoms, especially if diagnosis is before the age of six years. The reason for the improved prognosis is unclear because there are few specific interventions for children with FASD, but it may relate to improved understanding and appropriate expectations of the children by their caregivers and teachers.

Individuals with FASD may respond differently to stimulant medication than other children with ADHD. Specifically, children with FASD appear to have a differential response to methylphenidate and dexamphetamine. In a case series of 30 children with FASD and ADHD, 22% (of 23 children) responded to methylphenidate, while 79% (of 19 children) responded to dexamphetamine. Of the children given both medications, eight did not respond to methylphenidate but later responded to dexamphetamine, one child did not respond to dexamphetamine but later responded to methylphenidate, and three children did not respond to either medication. The apparently increased response rate to dexamphetamine may be explained by animal work showing that rats who were prenatally exposed to alcohol and had physical hyperactivity showed "hyperresponsiveness" to methylphenidate and that alcohol exposure acts on the D_1 dopamine receptors of the mesolimbic system, which is the site of action of dexamphetamine. Decreased effectiveness of methylphenidate in animal and human studies suggests that the front nigrostriatal pathway may not be the mechanism in patients with FASD and comorbid ADHD.

ADHD and FASD

There may be multiple pathways to the coexistence of ADHD symptoms and FASD, so there may be different subsets of ADHD and FASD. The relationship between ADHD and FASD may be coincidental because ADHD is a common disorder affecting up to 11% of children in the general population. Adults with ADHD are more likely to drink alcohol, thus pregnant women with ADHD who drink alcohol during pregnancy may genetically transmit ADHD to their offspring.

There may be common etiological pathways to ADHD and the behavioral phenotype of FASD. Alternatively, acquired ADHD secondary to prenatal alcohol exposure may be due to the effect of alcohol on the developing dopamine transmitter system. These two hypotheses are supported by changes in the neurochemistry seen in animal studies of fetal alcohol exposure in which deficits have been found in most neurotransmitter systems, including the dopaminergic, noradrenergic, serotonergic, cholinergic, glutaminergic, gamma aminobutyric acid (GABA)-ergic, and histaminergic systems. Deficits in noradrenergic and dopaminergic systems are the most likely ones to be related to the ADHD symptoms seen in animals with prenatal alcohol exposure. The D_1 receptors of the mesolimbic dopamine system tend to be affected by alcohol exposure more than other dopamine systems.

Some studies support the idea that ADHD in FASD is a particular clinical subtype with earlier onset, a different clinical and neuropsychologic profile, and a different response to psychostimulant medications. The Seattle Longitudinal Prospective Study suggests that infants with a history of prenatal alcohol exposure have an infant regulatory disorder and temperament disturbance which precede the diagnosis of ADHD. Research has shown that animals with prenatal alcohol exposure have an exaggerated response to psychostimulants, which is mediated by age, gender, and drug dosage. There is evidence suggesting that individuals with FASD and ADHD have a better response to dexamphetamine than methylphenidate. Patients, such as those with FASD, who have neurochemical or structural changes in the central nervous system are often hypersensitive to the effects and side effects of medication, and psychostimulant response in these patients may improve with age.

Adaptive behavior

Adaptive function is the ability to meet developmentally appropriate expectations of personal independence and social responsibility, including performance of everyday tasks, and adapt to changes in the environment. Adaptive behavior is affected in both FASD and ADHD. Using the Vinelands Adaptive Behavior Scale, three groups were compared, ie, children with heavy prenatal alcohol exposure, children with ADHD, and normally developing children. Children with prenatal alcohol exposure and children with ADHD had significantly lower scores on the communication domain than controls and, in the prenatal alcohol exposure group, age was negatively associated with score. Children in the prenatal alcohol exposure and ADHD groups had significantly lower scores on daily living skills, but the prenatal alcohol exposure group had significantly lower scores than the ADHD group. Children in the prenatal alcohol exposure and ADHD groups had significantly lower scores on socialization, but did not differ from each other. Again, age was negatively associated with the scores in the prenatal alcohol exposure group. Within the FASD group, children scored best in daily living skills and scored worst on socialization and communication domains. They demonstrated increasing adaptive behavior deficits with age. The children with ADHD had difficulty with socialization skills and their adaptive behavior skills improved with age. Overall, children in the prenatal alcohol exposure group were more likely than children in the ADHD and control groups to be rated as having inadequate adaptive skills. When analyzed with matched IQs, the prenatal alcohol exposure and ADHD groups did not differ from each other. For adaptive behavior skills, the differences between children with prenatal alcohol exposure and children with ADHD may be accounted for by IQ.

Executive function

Executive function is the higher order process involved in thought and action under conscious control, usually to achieve a goal. It involves planning, inhibition, working memory, organized speech, set-shifting, strategy employment, flexible thinking, and fluency. Executive function is probably mediated by the frontal cortex, and prenatal alcohol exposure may affect frontal cortex development. Neuropsychologic measures of executive function assess organization, planning, working memory, inhibition of inappropriate responses, and set-shifting.

The common symptoms of behavioral disinhibition and attention deficit in FASD and ADHD may be related to problems with executive function. There is evidence that executive function is a core deficit in FASD and ADHD, and neuroimaging shows that children with FASD and ADHD may have structural and functional abnormalities in the frontal-subcortical circuits, which are areas associated with executive function. Behavioral data also confirm that both populations have deficits in global adaptive abilities. There is conflicting evidence regarding executive function deficits in ADHD.

Nanson et al conducted a prospective cohort study comparing children with FAS or FAE with normal developing (control) children and children with attention deficit disorder (ADD) without FAS or FAE. Behavioral characteristics were similar between the FAS/FAE and ADD groups. There were no differences on parental rating for the two groups, suggesting it is difficult to distinguish between the two groups using traditional observational scales. The FAS/FAE group tended to have slower performance and was more likely to improve with practice than the ADD group. Unlike the ADD group, the FAS/FAE group was not able to trade off accuracy in favor of increased speed.

Coles et al compared children with prenatal alcohol exposure, children with ADHD without prenatal alcohol exposure, and control children with neither prenatal alcohol exposure nor ADHD. They used traditional behavioral and psychiatric measures of ADHD and externalizing behavior and neurocognitive measures of a four-factor model of attention. Children with FAS or FAE had similar global intellectual deficits to children with ADHD. Both groups had difficulty with sequential functioning, but the FAS/FAE group had greater difficulties on visual-spatial reasoning. The FAS/FAE group struggled on arithmetic, while ADHD group were poorer on reading/decoding. The FAS/FAE group had nonsignificant decreases in scores on reading/decoding. Both the FAS/FAE and ADHD groups had trouble with coding in the revised edition of the Wechsler Intelligence Scale for Children. The FAS/FAE children had problems with encoding on the second list of the paired-associate task and the number of categories completed on the Wisconsin Card Sorting Test (WCST). On behavioral measures, the ADHD group scored highest on the Child Behavior Checklist, the SNAP and the DISC (diagnostic interview schedule for children) interview items but the FAS/FAE group only differed from the control group on the attention score on the Child Behavior Checklist. On the Computer Performance Task, the ADHD group had poor speed and accuracy, slower reaction times, and more false alarms (associated with impulsivity). They also had fewer hits and more misses. However, there was a large dropout of children from the Computer Performance Task (60% of the ADHD group, 52% of the FAS/FAE group, and 43% of controls). Using the four-factor model of attention, the FAS/FAE group had problems with encoding and shift, while the ADHD group had difficulties with focus and sustain. The results of this study suggested that children with ADHD and FAS/FAE have unique attentional profiles, and thus the neurocognitive deficits may not be the same. The authors recommend that children with ADHD are best identified using behavior checklists and measures of the ability to focus and sustain attention, while children with FAS/FAE have deficits in visual-spatial skills, encoding of information, and flexibility in problem solving.

Vaurio et al examined executive function in children with heavy prenatal alcohol exposure, children with ADHD who were not exposed to prenatal alcohol, and children with neither ADHD nor prenatal alcohol exposure. The children with prenatal alcohol exposure performed worse than the ADHD group on letter fluency and category fluency. On Trail making Test-B, the prenatal alcohol exposure group differed significantly from the control group. The ADHD group did not differ significantly from the control group on this test. The prenatal alcohol exposure and ADHD groups had similar deficits on the WCST and both performed more poorly on letter fluency than category fluency. However, letter fluency was significantly poorer in the prenatal alcohol exposure group. In this study the prenatal alcohol exposure group performed better on the WCST than predicted by IQ but the ADHD group performed more poorly than predicted by IQ. This finding for the prenatal alcohol exposure group was in conflict with previous studies in which executive function deficits remained or worsened when IQ was controlled.

Summary

In summary, there is some evidence for distinguishing between children with FASD and children with ADHD. Using the four-factor model of attention it has been shown that children with FASD have difficulties with encoding and shift, while the children with ADHD have problems with focus and sustain. Other findings have not been consistently reproduced across studies and the usefulness of traditional behavioral observation scales for distinguishing between the two groups has not been proven. The main obstacles to comparison of study findings are the use of different inclusion criteria, definitions and outcome measures. In particular, published studies frequently include children with heavy prenatal alcohol exposure (variously defined) with or without confirmed FASD in one group.

Diagnosis of the Impulsive, Hyperactive, or Inattentive Child

The diagnosis of ADHD should only be made after a comprehensive assessment including a medical, developmental and psychosocial history, and examination. The DSM-IV criteria are the minimum requirement for a diagnosis of ADHD. ADHD is not an etiologic diagnosis, and assessment of the impulsive, hyperactive, or inattentive child should always include a thorough history and examination for potential causes, including alcohol exposure in pregnancy. Although enquiry regarding alcohol exposure in pregnancy should be routine, many health professionals do not ask.

Behavioral rating scales can provide useful information, in a standardized format, from multiple informants, and can be used to monitor response to treatment. Many measures are available, such as the Child Behavior Checklist, the Strength and Difficulties Questionnaires, and specific ADHD scales, eg, the Conners' rating scales. The Behavior Rating Inventory of Executive Function (BRIEF) is a useful tool for evaluating behavioral, social, and emotional aspects of executive functioning in children with FASD.

Standard criteria should be used for the diagnosis of FASD. The choice of diagnostic criteria will be determined by local guidelines and clinician preference. Assessment and diagnosis of FASD usually requires input from medical and allied health professionals due to the range of physical and neurologic structural and functional issues which can occur in FASD and are required to fulfill diagnostic criteria.

Treatment of ADHD in FASD

There is a paucity of high quality evidence assessing interventions for children with both FASD and ADHD. There are two very small, randomized, controlled trials which examine the use of stimulant medication. The first study compared methylphenidate with placebo (n = 4). Compared with placebo, methylphenidate improved hyperactivity and impulsivity symptoms but not attention. Adverse effects from the methylphenidate were reported for three of the four children, and one child had to discontinue methylphenidate 12 weeks into the trial due to excessive weight loss. In the second study, usual stimulant medication was compared with placebo (n = 12). Compared with placebo, stimulants improved hyperactivity symptoms but not attention. Psychopharmacologic agents have also been examined in retrospective and uncontrolled studies. In one study, stimulant medication improved hyperactivity and impulsivity scores, but inattention was less responsive to medication. In a retrospective study, there was a suggestion that children with ADHD and FASD had a preferential response to dexamphetamine. The role of atomoxetine is being assessed in two studies including one randomized controlled trial.

There is one study of behavioral or psychological intervention for children with FASD and ADHD symptoms, in which 23 children were randomized to receive attention process training or contact control sessions. The group receiving attention process training had significantly more improvement on measures of sustained attention and non-verbal reasoning ability than controls, but not on measures of executive function.

Because there is little evidence specific to the management of ADHD in FASD, the approach to intervention is mostly extrapolated from the ADHD literature. Multimodal therapy is the recommended treatment for ADHD in all age groups. This could include pharmacologic and behavioral interventions. The Multi-modal Treatment Study of Children with Attention-Deficit/Hyperactivity Disorder demonstrated that pharmacologic management was superior to an intensive behavioral intervention at a 14-months follow-up. Compared with pharmacologic management alone, combined pharmacologic and intensive behavioral interventions did not significantly improve core ADHD symptoms, but treatment outcomes were achieved with a significantly lower dose of medication in the combined treatment group than in the pharmacologic management group. The management plan should also take into consideration the comorbidities of ADHD and FASD.

Medication will not be needed for all individuals with ADHD and should only be used when the symptoms are pervasive across settings and are causing significant impairment in academic, social, or behavioral domains. Individuals receiving medication require regular review, at least six monthly. Medications for ADHD include stimulant (methylphenidate and dexamphetamine) and nonstimulant medications (eg, atomoxetine). Stimulant medications are thought to act by altering the availability of dopamine and noradrenaline, which influences behavior inhibition, impulse control, and attention. Clinicians should consider trialing dexamphetamine first, because there is some evidence suggesting that children with FASD have a preferential response to dexamphetamine over methylphenidate. Methylphenidate is available in immediate-release and extended-release formulations, but there is no evidence regarding the use of extended-release methylphenidate preparations in children with FASD. Atomoxetine is a nonstimulant medication which is classified as a noradrenaline reuptake inhibitor.[3] The evidence regarding atomoxetine use in FASD is pending. There is no evidence available regarding the use of other nonstimulant medications in FASD.

Conclusion

ADHD is the most frequent comorbidity of FASD but the exact relationship between the two entities is not well defined. There is some evidence that a specific clinical subtype of ADHD occurs in FASD, with earlier onset and a different response to medication. However, the relationship between ADHD and FASD may be coincidental, may reflect a common etiologic pathway, or may reflect the frequent genetic origin of ADHD and its prevalence in the general population. It is likely that a range of these etiologic factors account for ADHD in FASD, resulting in a heterogeneous population, which makes it difficult to replicate or generalize findings across studies.

Impairment of executive function may be a common underlying factor in ADHD and FASD but, using the four-factor model of attention, there is evidence of difference between these two groups. Children with FASD have difficulties with encoding and shift, and children with ADHD without FASD have problems with focus and sustain. If this difference is reproducible in large cohorts, then it may be useful for diagnosis in the clinical population.

There are clinical benefits to clarifying whether an individual has FASD because early diagnosis of FASD can ameliorate the secondary disabilities. There may be a differential medication response in individuals with ADHD who also have FASD, in particular a possible preferential response to dexamphetamine. However, the evidence to support treatments for ADHD in FASD is scarce.

There is a need for large, high quality studies examining the etiology, diagnosis, and interventions for ADHD in FASD because there is the potential to modify significantly the poor adult outcomes associated with the secondary disabilities. Agreement on the most appropriate diagnostic criteria and terminology for FASD and standardization of outcome measures would improve the translation of research findings into clinical practice. The development of effective interventions will be guided by improved understanding of the etiology of ADHD in FASD and the ability to diagnose FASD more accurately.

TIMELINE: FETAL ALCOHOL SPECTRUM DISORDERS

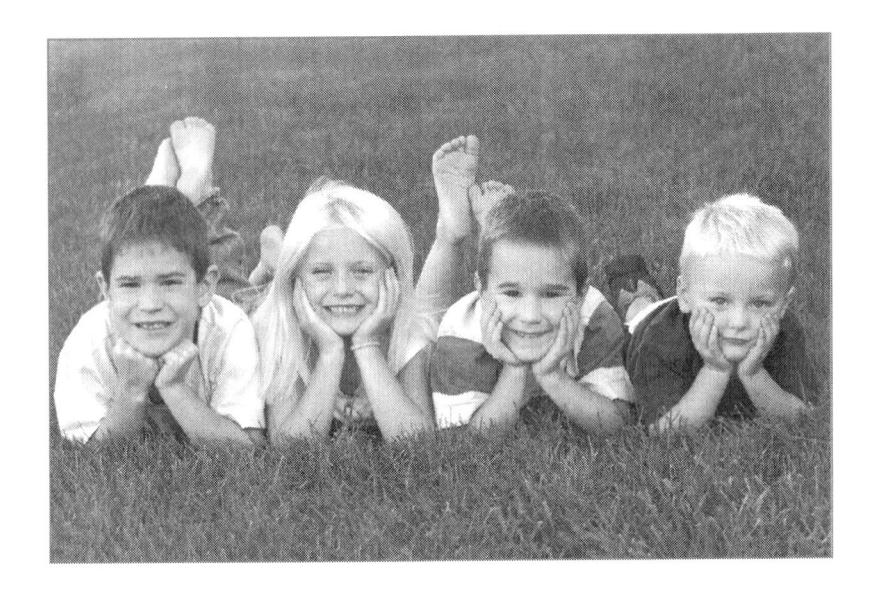

Yesterday

- Alcohol's ability to cause birth defects was recognized more than three decades ago by U.S. researchers, and it is now the leading known environmental teratogen (an agent capable of causing physical birth defects). In a 1981 advisory, the U.S. Surgeon General suggested that pregnant women should limit their alcohol intake – although no recommended level of intake was specified.

- Fetal alcohol syndrome (FAS) is one of the most serious consequences of heavy drinking during pregnancy. FAS is a devastating constellation of birth defects characterized by craniofacial malformations, neurological and motor deficits, intrauterine growth retardation, learning disabilities, and behavioral and social deficits.

- While the prevalence of FAS in the U.S. is between 0.5-2.0 cases per 1000 births, it is more common in other parts of the world. For example, in parts of South Africa where heavy drinking prevails, the incidence of FAS exceeds 60 cases per 1000 individuals.

It is estimated that for every child born with FAS, three additional children are born who may not have the physical characteristics of FAS but who, as a result of prenatal alcohol exposure, still experience neurobehavioral deficits that affect learning and behavior.

Today

- The umbrella term "Fetal Alcohol Spectrum Disorders (FASD)" is now used to characterize the full range of prenatal alcohol damage varying from mild to severe and encompassing a broad array of physical defects and cognitive, behavioral, and emotional deficits.

- The earliest stages of life are periods of great vulnerability to the adverse effects of alcohol. Embryonic and fetal development are characterized by rapid, but well-synchronized patterns of gene expression, which makes the embryo/fetus particularly vulnerable to harm from alcohol.

- Research shows that patterns of exposure known to place a fetus at greatest risk for FASD include drinking four or more drinks per occasion, and drinking more than seven drinks per week. The outcomes attributable to prenatal alcohol exposure for the children of women drinking in this manner include deficits in growth, behavior, and neurocognition, including deficits in arithmetic, language and memory, visual-spatial abilities, attention, and speed of information processing.

- Imaging and neurobehavioral research in individuals with FAS and FASD reveals that some brain regions appear to be most sensitive to prenatal alcohol while other areas apparently are spared adverse effects. Particularly vulnerable regions include the frontal cortex, hippocampus, corpus callosum, and components of the cerebellum, including the anterior vermis.

- Despite a number of prevention efforts, including point of sale warning signs and bottle labeling, national surveillance data indicate that in 2005, 12% of pregnant women admitted drinking alcohol in the previous month and 2% were binge drinking. Data from prenatal clinics and postnatal studies suggest that 20-30% of women drink at some time during pregnancy. A majority of women in the U.S. reduce or abstain from alcohol once pregnancy is recognized but almost half of pregnancies in the U.S. are unplanned. More than 12% of women who are not using contraception and are at risk of becoming pregnant drink at levels that exceed 7 drinks per week or 4 or more drinks per occasion.

- In a 2005 update of the Surgeon General's advisory of 1981, the U.S. Surgeon General advised pregnant women and women who may become pregnant to abstain from drinking alcohol to eliminate the chance of giving birth to a baby with FASD.

- The Surgeon General's 2005 advisory states:

    o A pregnant woman should not drink alcohol during pregnancy.

    o A pregnant woman who already has consumed alcohol during her pregnancy should stop in order to minimize further risk.

    o A woman who is considering becoming pregnant should abstain from alcohol.

    o Health professionals should routinely inquire about alcohol consumption by women of childbearing age, inform them of the risks of alcohol consumption during pregnancy, and advise them not to drink alcoholic beverages during pregnancy.

- Health professionals may offer brief office-based interventions to women at risk for an alcohol-exposed pregnancy or who are drinking during pregnancy, or may refer them to an alcohol treatment specialist. Women who continue to have difficulty refraining from alcohol after a brief intervention and those who are alcohol dependent should be referred to an alcohol treatment specialist.

A number of effective tools are available for assessment of at-risk drinking and intervention guidelines for women of childbearing age. Currently, the National Institute of Health (NIH) and other agencies and organizations recommend that primary care providers screen all women of childbearing age for alcohol use.

Tomorrow

- Ongoing NIH research seeks to find more effective ways to prevent and treat FASD. The broadest approach involves universal prevention measures targeted to the global community of men and women, and conveys general education on risks and information to abstain from alcohol in pregnancy.

- Current research also includes multilevel interventions involving case management of high risk individuals and brief interventions using motivational interviewing and community reinforcement.

- Screening, brief intervention, and referral for treatment (SBIRT) approaches have emerged as a significant tool for addressing alcohol and other substance use in primary and prenatal care settings. SBIRT has been endorsed by the NIH, the American College of Obstetricians and Gynecologists, and other federal agencies and professional societies.

Ongoing NIH research on computer-delivered brief interventions is beginning to show promising effects in the area of prenatal substance use, with early results suggesting that computer-delivered SBIRT may be implemented efficiently and at low cost in community settings.

- Other ongoing efforts to minimize the damage caused by prenatal alcohol exposure include studies of pharmacological intervention during pregnancy. This approach may be applicable when there is alcohol exposure before a woman recognizes that she is pregnant, or otherwise fails to stop drinking during the pregnancy.

- Early-stage clinical trials are underway to assess the ability of choline supplementation as well as several behavioral interventions to mitigate learning and behavioral deficits in children with FASD. In addition, basic science investigations are exploring a number of other potential therapeutic interventions, such as dietary choline supplementation during pregnancy to prevent FASD.

- Researchers are also using animal models of FASD to explore several promising approaches to reversing or ameliorating neurobehavioral deficits. For example, recent animal studies examining the effects of neonatal binge alcohol exposure on the performance of a motor task suggest that complex motor skill training may help reverse performance deficits resulting from such exposure.

The National Institute on Alcohol Abuse and Alcoholism (NIAAA) also seeks to launch an initiative to establish more precise estimates of FASD prevalence through creation of a standardized diagnostic system among affected children. While multiple studies designed to examine the risk factors for and effects of FASD have estimated the overall prevalence of FASD in the U.S., results of these studies suggest disparities due to relatively high rates of FASD in selected heavily drinking groups. There is a substantial need to determine a more accurate prevalence of FASD in broader communities exhibiting more variable risk.

BIBLIOGRAPHY

Centers for Disease Control and Prevention. *Fetal Alcohol Spectrum Disorders (FASDs)*. Retrieved April 10, 2014 from http://www.cdc.gov/ncbddd/fasd/index.html

Centers for Disease Control and Prevention. *Binge Drinking: A Serious, Under-Recognized Problem Among Women and Girls.* Retrieved April 10, 2014 from http://www.cdc.gov/vitalsigns/bingedrinkingfemale/

FASD Center. SAMHSA. *Fetal Alcohol Spectrum Disorders (FASDs).* Retrieved April 10, 2014 from http://www.fasdcenter.samhsa.gov/documents/WYNK_Effects_Fetus.pdf

National Center for Biotechnology Information. National Library of Medicine. National Institute of Health. *Dysregulation of microRNA Expression and Function Contributes to the Etiology of Fetal Alcohol Spectrum Disorders.* Retrieved April 10, 2014 from http://www.ncbi.nlm.nih.gov/pmc/articles/PMC3860419/

National Center for Biotechnology Information. National Library of Medicine. National Institute of Health. *Prenatal Alcohol Exposure and Cellular Differentiation.* Retrieved April 10, 2014 from http://www.ncbi.nlm.nih.gov/pmc/articles/PMC3860417/

National Center for Biotechnology Information. National Library of Medicine. National Institute of Health. *Distinguishing between attention-deficit hyperactivity and fetal alcohol spectrum disorders in children: clinical guidelines.* Retrieved April 10, 2014 from http://www.ncbi.nlm.nih.gov/pmc/articles/PMC2938300/

National Institute of Health. Cognitive changes may be only sign of fetal alcohol exposure. Retrieved April 10, 2014 from http://www.nih.gov/news/health/jul2012/nichd-23.htm

National Institute on Alcohol Abuse and Alcoholism. National Institute of Health. *Fetal Alcohol Spectrum Disorders.* Retrieved April 10, 2014 from http://pubs.niaaa.nih.gov/publications/arh40/118-126.htm

National Institute on Alcohol Abuse and Alcoholism. National Institute of Health. *Research: Fetal Alcohol Spectrum Disorders.* Retrieved April 10,

2014 from http://niaaa.nih.gov/research/major-initiatives/fetal-alcohol-spectrum-disorders

National Institute on Alcohol Abuse and Alcoholism. National Institute of Health. *Maternal Risk Factors for Fetal Alcohol Spectrum Disorders: Not As Simple As It Might Seem.* Retrieved April 10, 2014 from http://pubs.niaaa.nih.gov/publications/arh341/15-26.htm

National Institute on Alcohol Abuse and Alcoholism. National Institute of Health. *Fetal Alcohol Exposure.* Retrieved April 10, 2014 from http://www.niaaa.nih.gov/alcohol-health/fetal-alcohol-exposure

National Library of Medicine. National Institute of Health. *Fetal Alcohol Spectrum Disorders.* Retrieved April 10, 2014 from http://www.nlm.nih.gov/medlineplus/fetalalcoholspectrumdisorders.html

National Library of Medicine. National Institute of Health. *Fetal Alcohol Syndrome.* Retrieved April 10, 2014 from http://www.nlm.nih.gov/medlineplus/ency/article/000911.htm

National Library of Medicine. National Institute of Health. *Alcohol and pregnancy.* Retrieved April 10, 2014 from http://www.nlm.nih.gov/medlineplus/ency/article/007454.htm

Report. National Institute of Health. *Fetal Alcohol Spectrum Disorders.* Retrieved April 10, 2014 from http://report.nih.gov/NIHfactsheets/ViewFactSheet.aspx?csid=27

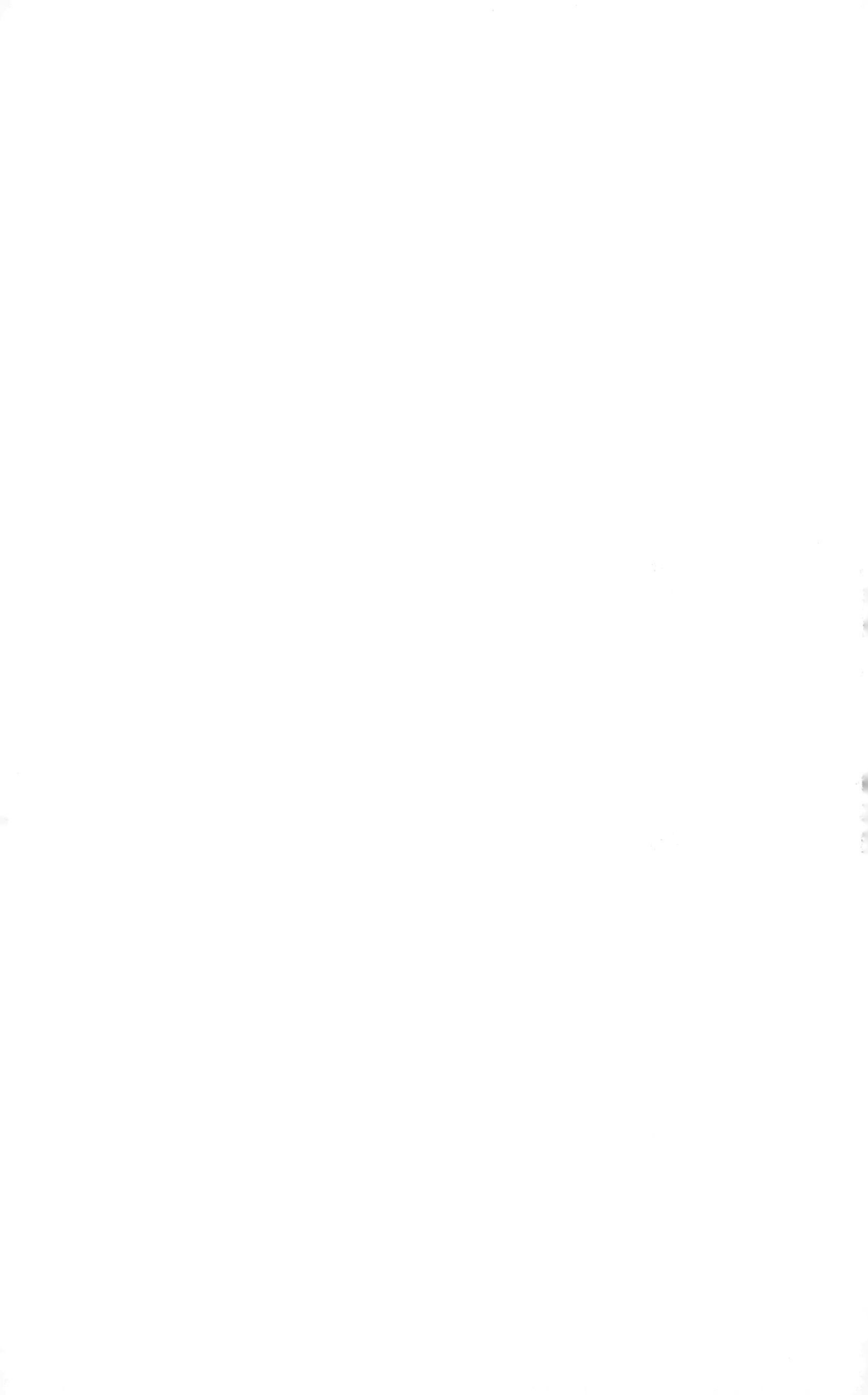

Made in the USA
Lexington, KY
06 July 2014